THE LITTLE BLACK BOOK OF WORKOUT MOTIVATION

Michael Matthews

OCULUS PUBLISHERS

Cover Designed by Winning Edits (*www.winningedits.com*)

Edited by Winning Edits (*www.winningedits.com*)

Published by Oculus Publishers, Inc. (*www.oculuspublishers.com*)

Visit the author's website:
www.muscleforlife.com

Praise for
The Little Black Book

"Matthews has hit it out of the ballpark with this *Little Black Book*. This is not your typical 'rah rah' self-help book full of tired clichés. It's a unique, meticulously researched and compelling combination of storytelling, science, and practical tools and takeaways."

> —Ben Greenfield, CEO of Kion & *New York Times* best-selling author of *Beyond Training: Mastering Endurance, Health & Life*

"This is a good, helpful, important book that establishes Mike as the Jordan Peterson of fitness. Any person who wants to train more effectively will benefit from reading it between sets, and will never give a copy to the guys he wants to beat."

> —Mark Rippetoe, author of *Starting Strength: Basic Barbell Training and Practical Programming for Strength Training*

"Matthews is a master of the mental side of fitness, so you'll finish this book fired up to get to work—and, more importantly, with the practical tools you need to start your journey successfully."

> —Alex Hutchinson, author of the *New York Times* best seller *Endure: Mind, Body, and the Curiously Elastic Limits of Human Performance*

"Read this book and absorb and apply its wisdom, and your life will get better. It's that simple."

> —Mark Divine, founder of SEALFIT and *New York Times* best-selling author of *The Way of the SEAL, Unbeatable Mind,* and *8 Weeks to SEALFIT*

"I love Mike's writing. Backed by a sh*t ton of research, crystal clear, and always actionable."

> —Noah Kagan, cofounder of Sumo.com and AppSumo.com

"The word 'goal' should be a verb, because a goal without action is just a dream. *The Little Black Book of Workout Motivation* provides all the tools you need to turn your goals into reality—and to never, ever feel 'stuck' again."

> —Jeff Haden, Inc. contributing editor and author of *The Motivation Myth: How High Achievers Really Set Themselves Up to Win*

"This book will challenge you, it will make you think, it will force you to go outside your comfort zone. It will help you build much more than motivation, but an inner drive to succeed so you can weather any storm."

> —Marc Perry, CSCS, CPT, Founder and CEO of BuiltLean

"Mike has already taught us how to be bigger, leaner and stronger—and it works. Now he teaches how to be BETTER in all areas of life. A concise, indispensable guide to fitness and effectiveness."

—Strauss Zelnick, "America's fittest CEO"

"In the charlatan-packed world of the fitness industry, Mike Matthews is a breath of fresh air. This book will inspire you and inform you with quality, applicable information that isn't biased. If you want to improve your physique and your life, do yourself a favor and read *The Little Black Book*."

—Sal Di Stefano, cohost of top-ranked fitness and health podcast *Mind Pump*

"Mike Matthews delivers another gem. *The Little Black Book* is chock-full of unbiased, evidence-based knowledge that you should not live without. A must-read."

—Adam Schafer, cohost of top-ranked fitness and health podcast *Mind Pump*

Dedication

To everyone who reads my crap, some of which I'm proud of, and some of which, well, you know, let's just leave it at "crap."

Seriously, though, I love you guys and gals and hope you find this book helpful.

Table of Contents

Who Is Mike Matthews, and Why Should I Care?

"Moderation is a fatal thing.
Nothing succeeds like excess."
—Oscar Wilde

'm Mike, and I believe that every person can achieve the body of their dreams. My mission is to give everyone that opportunity by providing time-proven, evidence-based advice on how to build muscle, lose fat, and get and stay healthy.

I've been training for more than a decade now. In that time, I've read thousands of pages of scientific literature and tried just about every type of workout program, diet regimen, and supplement you can imagine. At this point, I can confidently say that while I don't know everything, I know what works and what doesn't.

Like most guys who get into weightlifting, I had no clue what I was doing when I started out. I turned to fitness magazines for help, which had me spending a couple hours in the gym every day and wasting hundreds of dollars on pills and powders each month. This went on for years, and I jumped from diet to diet, workout program to workout program, and supplement to supplement, only to make mediocre progress and eventually get stuck in a rut.

I then turned to personal trainers for guidance, but they just had me do more of the same. After spending many thousands of dollars with them, I still hadn't gained any muscle or strength to speak of, and still had no idea what to do with my diet and nutrition to reach my goals. I liked working out too much to quit, but I wasn't happy with my body, and didn't know what I was doing wrong.

Here's a picture of me about seven years into my journey:

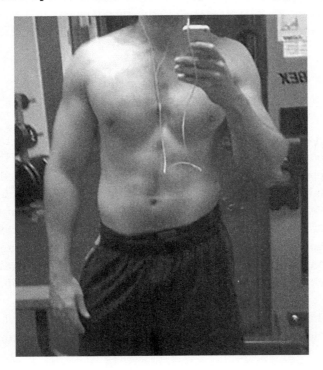

I didn't look bad by any means, but that's not exactly what you'd expect from fifteen hundred-plus hours of working out with no extended breaks.

I finally decided that something had to change, and I knew that I needed to start with learning the actual physiology of muscle growth and fat loss. So I threw the magazines away, fired the trainers, got off the internet forums, and searched out the work of top strength and bodybuilding coaches, talked to scores of natural bodybuilders, and started reading scientific papers.

Several months later, a clear picture was beginning to emerge.

The real science of getting into incredible shape is very simple—much simpler than the fitness industry want us to believe. It flies in the face of a lot of the crap we read in most books and magazines, and see on YouTube and in the gym.

For example . . .

- You don't need supplements to build a great physique.
- You don't need to constantly change up your workout routine to "confuse" your muscles.
- You don't need to "eat clean" to get and stay lean.
- You don't need to stop eating carbs and sugars to lose weight.
- You don't need to eat small meals every few hours to "boost your metabolism."
- You don't need to grind out hours and hours of boring cardio every week to shed ugly belly fat and get a shredded six-pack.

As a result of what I had learned, I completely changed my approach to eating and exercising, and my body responded in ways I couldn't believe. My strength skyrocketed. My muscles started growing again. My energy levels went through the roof. And here's the kicker: I was spending less time in the gym, and eating foods I actually liked.

Here's how my body has changed since:

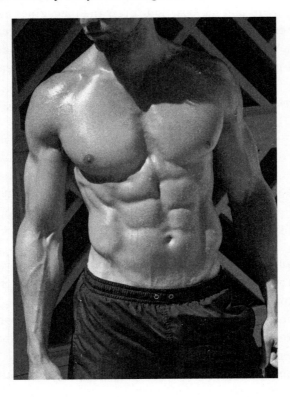

It shouldn't have taken as long to get here as it did, but hey, better late than never, right?

Along the way, my friends and family noticed how my body was changing and began asking for advice. I became their coach. I took "hardgainers" and put thirty pounds on them in a year, took people who were absolutely baffled as to why they couldn't lose weight and stripped piles of fat off them (and added muscle to their frames as well), and took people in their forties, fifties, and sixties who believed their hormones and metabolisms were beyond repair and helped them get into the best shape of their lives.

A couple years later, my "clients" (I never asked for money—I just had them come train with me) started urging me to write a book. I dismissed the idea at first, but began to warm up to it. "What if I'd had such a book when I started training?" I thought. It would have saved me who knows how much time, money, and frustration, and I would have built the body of my dreams a lot faster. I also enjoyed helping people with what I had learned, and if I were to write a book and it became popular, what if I could help thousands or even hundreds of thousands of people?

That gave me a wild hair, and so I wrote *Bigger Leaner Stronger* and published it in January 2012. It sold maybe twenty copies in the first month, but within a couple months, sales were growing, and I began receiving emails from readers with high praise. I was floored. I started making notes on how I could improve the book based on feedback, and outlined ideas for several other books that I could write.

Fast forward to today, and I've now published a number of books, including a diet and exercise book for women (*Thinner Leaner Stronger*) and a flexible dieting cookbook (*The Shredded Chef*). Altogether, my books have sold over a million copies, and my work has been featured in a number of publications like *Men's Health*, *Muscle & Strength*, *Elle*, *Esquire*, and more.

More importantly, every day I get scores of emails and social media messages from readers who are thankful for my work and blown away by the results they're seeing. They're just as shocked as I was years ago when I first discovered just how straightforward and enjoyable getting fit and healthy can really be.

This is why I continue to write books and articles, record podcasts and YouTube videos, and generally do everything I can to be as helpful as I can to as many people as I can. It's motivating to see the impact I'm having on people's lives, and I'm incredibly inspired by the dedication and determination of so many of my readers and followers. You guys and gals rock.

I also have bigger ambitions that I want to realize.

First, I want to help a million people get fit and healthy. "Help a million people" just has a sexy ring to it, don't you think? It's a big goal, but I think I can do it. This goes beyond merely making people look hotter too. I want to make a dent in the alarming downward trends we're seeing here in the West, in particular, in people's overall physical and mental health and performance, and I think helping people get strong and fit is a great way to do that.

Second, I want to lead the fight against mainstream health and fitness pseudoscience and BS. Unfortunately, this space is full of misinformation, disinformation, idiots, liars, and hucksters, and I want to do something about it. I'd like to become known as the go-to guy for practical, easy-to-understand advice grounded in real science and results.

Third, I want to help reform the sport supplements industry. The pill and powder pushers rely on all types of scams to foist their junk products on unwitting consumers. They use fancy-sounding-but-worthless ingredients; they cut their products with junk fillers like flour and unnecessary amino acids; they use tiny, ineffective doses of otherwise good ingredients ("pixie dusting") and hide it with the notorious "proprietary blend"; and they rely on fake science, overhyped marketing claims, and steroid-fueled meatheads to convince people they have the "secret sauce."

I hope you enjoy this book, and I hope it helps you reach your health and fitness goals faster.

Mike Matthews
Vienna, Virginia
April 6, 2018

The Reinvention of Jennifer

When a great ship is in harbor and moored, it is safe.
But that is not what great ships are built for.
—Dr. Clarissa Estes

"I set goals all the time, but I just can't make myself do all the things I need to do."

Jennifer has to force the sentence out, shaking her head.

She's ashamed with more than the words—she's ashamed with herself. Many people wouldn't understand why. She's thirty-two years old, attractive, and living well by most standards. She has a good job, she gets stuff done, and she has close friends who admire her. Some even say they wish they were her.

Yet here she is, fighting back tears because, at bottom, she's afraid. Not of failure, humiliation, or hardship, but of remaining stuck in a state of quiet, mediocre desperation, of never quite discovering what she's truly capable of.

"Why do you think that is?" I ask.

She looks away for a moment. We're on a pier on a windswept beach in Florida, and whitecaps are rushing in toward throngs of laughing children at the shore, crashing and fizzing around their skittering feet.

"I don't know. Maybe I'm just too lazy. Or maybe I just don't really care enough—"

I interrupt her. "It's normal to feel like that, but you're wrong. And I can prove it."

Three months later, Jennifer and I had a very different discussion. It was a celebration. She had melted nearly twenty pounds of fat off her body, gained a considerable amount of muscle in the "right places," and realized that she did have the power to transform her body. Her newfound gumption was rippling out into other areas of her life as well. For the first time in a long time, she felt unstuck.

How did I help her do this, and how might I be able to help you do the same?

This book is the answer. In it, I'm going to share with you exactly what I shared with Jennifer, and I hope that it can you help you in the same way it helped her.

This book is for people who want to be better than they are right now.

People who have a vision for their bodies and lives, and who are driven to break free of artificial limitations and be better, live better, and fulfill their true potential.

It's for people who hate feeling like they're moving in slow motion, who don't want to surrender to the deadening effects of exhaustion and inertia, and who want to develop the physical, emotional, and spiritual strength and energy needed to look and live vigorously.

It's for people who are driven to heal what's unhealthy, fix what's broken, and improve what's lacking, and who believe that no matter the circumstances, something can always be done about it.

It's for people who want to feel in control of their destinies and who want to reach their graves with stories worth telling.

That said, this book isn't for everyone.

It's not for people who are happy coasting on cozy goals and pleasures, and who are contented with merely buying and consuming things that others create.

It's not for people who want to languish in a fool's paradise and avoid the ground truth about positive change—although ultimately rewarding, the process is often hard, draining, boring, and even depressing.

It's not even necessarily for people who are "unmotivated," because in my experience, this is very difficult to change. Instead, this book is for people who have a burning desire to be, do, and have more, and who could use some help with the "how."

As a best-selling author and coach, I've worked with thousands of smart, capable, hard-working people like Jennifer who have struggled to make "simple" changes in their lives. They want to stop doing harmful things like overspending or overeating, or want to start or keep doing positive things like exercising or educating themselves. While they generally know what they have to do, "life" just keeps finding a way to thwart their efforts. Sometimes it flashes shiny objects to distract, sometimes it offers ill-fated "shortcuts" to discourage, and sometimes it crosses tracks to derail. And in too many cases, life wins. It knocks too many people down too many times, who then brand themselves failures and stop trying to get up.

You probably know what I'm talking about. We've all been

there. And we're all wrong. What we've done or failed to do doesn't forever determine who we are or will be. In fact, I believe that we have no idea what we can really do. We may never find out, either—there may always be another level—but striving to reach the top is the most rewarding adventure life has to offer.

I wrote this book to help you in that quest to seize the experience of being alive. This is a journey that many thousands have already taken, and that is open to all. It requires no great talent, intelligence, or blessings, only the will to discover the path and walk it.

To help you do this, this book is going to focus less on particular methods than on time-proven principles, because blind adherence to processes without an understanding of the underlying rules results in rigid, maladaptive behaviors and attitudes. It's easy to mistakenly believe that because someone before us succeeded by doing A, B, and C, we can do the same and experience the same results. This type of thinking is seductive because it appeals to the parts of us that are timid and lazy, but it also conveniently ignores the fact that no two products of nature are ever exactly the same. Circumstances never repeat themselves exactly.

On the other hand, by learning to think in a principled way and exploring the reasoning behind those principles, we can successfully choose, discard, and even invent methods accordingly.

This book isn't going to be a clinical discussion of the science of motivation. Much of what you're going to learn is based on decades of scientific research, but both of us know that books like that don't work. People do. And what makes people work are ideas worth working for, and a clear understanding of what to do and how to do it. Intellectualizing isn't enough. We must reach the level of conviction before we can truly internalize and embody new ideals and behaviors.

That's why I want you to test this stuff out and even challenge it as you move through the book. You won't need any new skills—you already know how to focus, write things down, make decisions, and take action—and you'll probably find that many of the things you've already been doing instinctively and intuitively are right.

In this book, I will expose many of the prevailing myths about "motivation," including why goal setting, "positive thinking," and playing to your natural inclinations and disinclinations aren't enough to win in a world full of honeypots, deadfalls, and dead ends.

For at least the last couple of decades, many brilliant people have been working tirelessly not to advance our general knowledge, judgment, or capabilities, but to convince us to buy more things we don't need, consume more poisonous foods and vacuous entertainment, and conform our thoughts and beliefs to a cultural hive mind that worships whatever feels right.

And so it's no surprise that we have a dysfunctional "normal" where most people are comfortably numb. They've resigned themselves to what they believe they can and can't do and change, and have accepted the rules and restrictions dinned into them since childhood. According to various surveys and studies, they're on average twenty-three pounds overweight, they do just three hours of real work and watch five hours of TV per day, and they're over $130,000 in debt with less than $1,000 in savings. They sit. They eat. They watch. And they die.

Somewhere along the way, though, they'll wonder what happened and whom to blame for their misfortunes. "It's not your fault," the psychosocial tastemakers will coo. "You're not responsible for your condition. You're a victim of your circumstances." Yes, something in them will say, that feels good. That must be right. And then the power dive begins.

To master motivation, then, you have to get radically honest with yourself and the reality you face, and go far beyond what you find familiar and comfortable, because as unnatural as modern living is, it isn't the real enemy.

What's the real enemy? The part of us that clings to the default and status quo and recoils from anything it deems dangerous, difficult, or different. This is the only thing that can stop us from transforming who we are into who we want to be.

This is the part of us that says there are things we just can't do, boundaries we can't overstep, and rules we can't break, and we buy into it because it gives us a false sense of security. Even if we're completely dissatisfied with our everyday existence, at least we know the lay of the land and what to expect.

This is the part of us that says we should just do whatever makes us happy. If something is instinctive and spontaneous, then it must be right.

This is also the part of us that rejects golden opportunities to advance and evolve because they seem strange or dubious. And so we shy away, because we've been conditioned to fear the unknown.

We submit to these genetic and social instructions because they're the well-worn paths of least resistance. Even if we're adrift in the tides of unknowable forces, at least we aren't alone. Even if we're wearing blinders, at least they're hiding things we don't want to see.

By the end of this book, you will never again wonder what it takes to stay motivated to build the body and life of your dreams.

You will be inspired by compelling ideas and stories, and you will be empowered with a set of reliable, science-based principles, strategies, and habits that have been shown to work with a broad range of personalities to produce sustainable, long-term results.

This isn't to say that you will become "superhuman," or even that you need to. Ironically, most of the wildly successful people I've known don't see themselves as all that special. They experience disappointments, decision traps, and uncertainty, just like everyone else. They struggle with procrastination, habit making and breaking, and second guessing, and often more than others because they're so dedicated to pushing their limits. They've just learned to deal with these more unsavory aspects of life differently than most, and you can too.

This is going to feel unnatural and awkward at first, because, well, it is. You're going to bumble and stumble. You're going to slip and fall. And sometimes, you're even going to want to give up. All that is totally normal. Welcome to the club. This is the process. This is how you transform. I've been there myself, and so has every other person I've ever known who has escaped the strike zone of a "normal" life that makes no difference to anyone and changes nothing.

Armed with the information you're going to learn in the pages ahead, you're going to start living life with more energy, enthusiasm, and nerve. You're going to develop a new paradigm for interacting with yourself and your environment. And if you really take these lessons to heart, you might just enter a transformative period of your life and discover that you're capable of far more than you ever thought possible.

So, here's what I want you to do right now: read the next two chapters today. Yes, today. I know you're busy and you have lots to do, but jump in and commit, and in just fifteen minutes or so, your transformation will have officially begun.

Excellence can be yours. Your best body and life ever await. Just turn the page.

How to Use This Book

"If you have everything under control, you're not moving fast enough."
—Mario Andretti

Many people struggle to realize their ambitions because they spend too much time thinking and too little time doing and looking.

They formulate perfectly reasonable decisions to do perfectly wonderful things based on perfectly accurate observations, and then start the process of self-sabotage: thinking.

I'm pretty busy right now. Maybe this isn't the right time.

I'm probably too young/old/uneducated/uncreative/uncredentialed/pessimistic/etc.

What if this doesn't work? What if I fail? What will people think?

It's not long before those who survive this initial bombardment of weaponized head trash and actually get started have to endure another wave of assault.

This doesn't feel right.

I don't think I'm ready for this.

This isn't very fun.

The ranks are thinned again, leaving fewer people still in the fray. Before long, another barrage is unleashed.

Do I really care about this?

I'm exhausted.

Maybe I'm not good enough after all.

More hopes and dreams are blown into smithereens as the cannons are reloaded, and those still standing wonder when the offensive will relent.

For many people, it never does, but that doesn't necessarily stop them. Abraham Lincoln suffered from spells of severe depression throughout his entire adult life. For many years, John D. Rockefeller fretted endlessly about his company and didn't get a single night of solid sleep. "All the fortune that I have made has not served to compensate for the anxiety of that period," he later said. George Eliot, whose opus *Middlemarch* has been called the greatest novel in the English language, was so self-conscious of her writing that she used a male pseudonym and dreaded every submission to her publisher.

I wish I could say that we will have it better—that we won't have to weather our own storms—but it's simply not true. We will have to jump into the trenches like everyone else if we want to get anywhere, and the farther we want to go, the deeper we will have to venture into the labyrinth. That doesn't mean we have to become a casualty, though.

If we can do just one brutally simple thing well, then no amount of psychological and emotional trauma can put us down. If we can truly embrace this one little thing, then we can even learn to tune out the treacherous voices in our heads and inoculate ourselves against their poison.

This little thing is *action*. By staying in motion, the roots of doubt and despair can't take hold and ensnare us. By doing things, we can't be stopped by thinking things.

That doesn't mean we shouldn't plan, deliberate, and reflect, of course. We must be able to assess reality and deal with it as it is, not as we wish it were. It means that we shouldn't feed the trolls that live in the shadowy recesses of our minds.

That's why this book is going to ask you to do more than just read and think. Although it has "motivation" in its title, it's meant to do more than make you feel something, because that's never enough. As the old Chinese proverb goes, "Tell me, I'll forget; show me, I'll remember; involve me, I'll understand."

As you'll see, every chapter is going to end with a "Do This Now" section that is going to have you put what you just learned through its paces. This way, you can quickly see what will help you and what won't.

All you need to do these exercises is some paper (or a notebook) and a pen. You can also find them, along with chapter summaries, in the free bonus material available at www.workoutmotivationbook.com/bonus.

If I've done my job well and you follow my instructions, then you will be closer to the person you want to be and the life you want to live by the time you finish this book. How much closer will depend on many things, not the least of which will be how much action you're willing to take.

So let's begin, shall we?

CULTIVATING THE RIGHT MINDSET

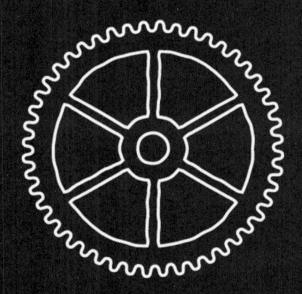

CHAPTER ONE

The Little Big Things About Building a Better You

"We who cut mere stones must always be envisioning cathedrals."
—*Quarry Worker's Creed*

People didn't get why Dan was doing it.

Why was he pouring so much time and energy into working out? Why was it so important to him?

Was it narcissism? Had he fallen in love with his reflection?

Maybe it was insecurity? Was he wrestling with an inferiority complex?

Or was it something darker, like self loathing? Was he unable to accept himself the way he was?

They were all missing the point.

Dan didn't train to feel vainglorious, paper over shortcomings, or punish himself. He did it because it gave him more than a better body. It gave him a better life.

When Dan first reached out to me, he was in a bad way. He was thirty-seven years old, thirty-something pounds overweight, and frustrated and confused. Name a diet, and he had tried it. He had run the gauntlet of popular exercise programs without much to show for it. You don't want to know how much money he had wasted on clueless trainers.

Dan was ready to resign himself to the apparent reality that it was just too late. For one reason or another—hormones, metabolism, stress, voodoo hexes—it appeared that his opportunity to get into great shape had come and gone without even a whisper.

He was wrong, of course. He just needed the right diet and exercise principles and systems. At first, he was skeptical of my advice. He thought it was too simple, that there was no way you could control your body's fat-burning and muscle-building machinery that easily. "Give me four weeks," I said, "and if you're not absolutely floored by the results, I'll pay you $1,000."

A month later, he was in disbelief. For the first time in his adult life, he was seeing real, measurable changes in how he looked and felt, and he was doing it without starving himself, following a restrictive diet, or eating foods he didn't like. He could do this for the rest of his life, he realized. That was several years ago, and Dan hasn't stopped. In fact, he's now in better shape than his college days. Twenty-year-old Dan wishes he had forty-year-old Dan's body.

He also realized that his workouts build more than muscle. They build character.

They teach us how to have the courage to commit to goals.

They teach us how to create purpose and meaning.

They teach us how to stop making excuses and finding reasons to fail.

They teach us how to stop being a victim and take responsibility for ourselves.

They teach us how to stop chasing magic bullets and quick fixes and embrace the process.

They teach us how to get gritty and push through pain and adversity.

They teach us how to value long-term satisfaction over immediate gratification.

At bottom, working out teaches us a very powerful lesson:

If we have the power to change our bodies, we have the power to change our lives.

That's why we train.

We train because fitness is one of those special things in life that you can't buy, steal, or fake. There aren't any rewards for complaining or failing, and fitness doesn't care about your opinions or feelings.

You have to give something to get something. You can't slide by on bullshit. It's called "working out," after all, and for good reason. You either do the work, and transform your body, or you don't.

This is a valuable lesson to learn, because it's a metaphor for something bigger. No matter what you're facing in life, you have two choices: you can put in the work or get put in your place.

Nature smiles at the economic, political, and social institutions we erect to try to change this. Let's not forget that not so long ago, our forebears had to chase, fight, and kill just to survive. They expected hardship. They were willing to face the worst. They embraced the fact that the universe, in all its apparent tranquility, is a carefully balanced chaos of forces that we barely understand.

We, on the other hand, have it easy. And that makes it easy

to go soft, lose perspective, and be lulled into idleness.

Working out is something of an inoculation against this. It's a tribute to the primacy of effort. A reminder that unless we're willing to work for them, "secrets" will never work. Reading books or blogs may supply pieces to the puzzle, but we still have to roll up our sleeves and figure out how they all fit together. All that can point us to the work, but then we have to do it.

If you find this discouraging, you're looking at it wrong. Groping for shortcuts is discouraging. Stumbling around in the dark, anxiously turning over rocks in search of arcana is discouraging. Waiting for lightning to strike your bottle is discouraging.

On the other hand, "donning the yoke" can be incredibly encouraging. Yes, it's bulky and uncomfortable, and yes, it demands toil and sweat, but it also promises a return on your efforts. You may not always get the prize you want, but you never leave empty-handed.

This makes the gym a lot more than a place to move, grunt, and sweat.

It's a microcosm where we can make contact with the deeper parts of ourselves—our convictions, fears, habits, and anxieties. It's an arena where we can confront these opponents head-on and prove that we have what it takes to vanquish them.

It's a setting where we can test the stories we tell ourselves. It calls on us to demonstrate how we respond to the greater struggles of life—adversity, pain, insecurity, stress, weakness, and disadvantage—and, in some ways, who we really are. In this way, the gym is a training and testing ground for the body, mind, and soul.

The conflicts we learn to endure in the gym empower us in our daily lives as well. The concentration, discipline, and resilience carry over. The way to do anything is, at bottom, the way to do everything.

The gym is also a source of learning, because it calls on us to constantly attempt new things. It's a forum where questions are at least as important as answers, and it cultivates what scientists call a "growth mindset" by teaching us that our abilities can be developed through dedication and hard work—a worldview that's essential for great accomplishment.

The gym is practical, too, not idealistic. It's a laboratory open to any and all ideas and methodologies, and it gives clear, unqualified feedback: they either work or they don't.

In short, the gym can be so much more than merely a place to work out. It can be a refuge from the chaos around us, a world of our own that we create to satisfy dreams and desires.

The gym can also provide us with something missing from so many people's lives: principles, values, and standards to live by. In short, a game worth playing.

Without a game worth playing, nothing else really matters. Life becomes a daisy chain of random events that happen to us, accidentally rather than intentionally, without rhyme or reason, direction or meaning.

It doesn't have to be like this, though. Fate has dealt us a hand, but we get to choose how we play it.

This is one of the many reasons to love fitness: It has purpose, order, and significance. It's an outlet for integrity, intention, and excellence. It fosters community, commitment, and a clear focus on worthwhile results. The type of results that bespeak prized virtues like discipline, patience, work ethic, self-respect, and passion. The type that speak louder than words and posture.

The fitness game goes deeper than that too. It's a "meta-game," so to speak, because if you have what it takes to conquer your psychology and physiology, then you might just have what it takes to reach out into the world and conquer a whole lot more. In short, the better you get at the fitness game, the better prepared you'll be for every other game you might want to play.

Whose story better exemplifies that than Arnold Schwarzenegger's?

Born in Austria in 1947 to an alcoholic ex-Nazi who beat him as a child, forced him to do sit-ups to earn breakfast, and ridiculed his boyhood dreams of becoming a bodybuilder, Arnold's rise to fame and fortune was a masterclass in self-determination.

As a kid, Arnie promised himself that he would leave Austria and make something more of his life, and he found inspiration in the most unlikely of places: a magazine article on the iconic bodybuilder turned movie star Reg Park.

Arnold's imagination soared. He envisioned himself becoming the most muscular man in the world, and then making blockbuster movies and enjoying million-dollar paydays. That's exactly what he would do, he told himself, and so he began training his body.

His friends were amused. "Come on, you're dreaming," they would say. "Give it up." His father was harsher. He said that such fantasies were embarrassing, and arranged for Arnold to be shipped off to the military at eighteen, where there would be no time or equipment for bodybuilding. Or so he thought.

Arnold resolved to do whatever it would take to make his daydream a reality, so, after long, grueling days of running, crawling, marching, shooting, and soldiering, when everyone else was literally collapsing from exhaustion, he worked out, sometimes for hours, using chairs, benches, bars and whatever else was at hand.

As usual, Arnold's peers lampooned his antics. They saw a useless fool trying to build castles in the sky, but Arnie wasn't fazed. He was determined to break through, no matter what it took. Reaching his goal of being a world champion became his singular focus in life.

Arnold's first chance to make a splash in the bodybuilding scene came when he was invited to compete in the junior Mr. Europe competition in Stuttgart, Germany. There was a problem, though: it would require that he abandon basic training and face severe consequences upon his return. Night after night he turned it over in his mind. Was he really ready to go to jail to compete in a bodybuilding show? Was all this really just a crazy delusion?

No, it wasn't, he decided. Reg Park did it, and he could too. When he closed his eyes at night, he saw himself standing on the stage, triumphant, just like his idol, and knew that he had to go. So he snuck out of the base, stowed away on a freight train, rode for twenty-six hours, borrowed another competitor's trunks (he didn't own any), shuffled onto stage, and awkwardly presented his physique to the skeptical judges and crowd.

And he won first place.

This was a watershed moment. It gave Arnold something tangible to hang his hat on. It proved that maybe he wasn't so foolish after all.

But there was a problem—he was also still enlisted in the Austrian army. Furthermore, after unsuccessfully trying to sneak back into his barracks, he was castigated by his superiors and thrown into solitary confinement.

After cooling down, though, the officers wanted to know if it was true: did Arnold actually win the show? Indeed he did, he explained, and it was all thanks to the rigors of their training, he added, playing up to his seniors. As men who valued discipline above all, they accepted the invitation to share in his victory and even began presenting Arnold as a model recruit.

From here, Arnold continued to build, mold, and sculpt his body while completing his stint in the army. He then took the bodybuilding scene by storm, and in just a few short years, had not only mounted its highest pedestal, but helped transform the sport from an obscure, low-rent hobby into a glamorous celebration of the physical aesthetic.

Becoming the best bodybuilder in the world was only the first phase of his plan, though. The next domain to conquer was the silver screen, so Arnie went west, only to be met with scorn. The awkward accent, the bulging muscles, the weird name—none of it worked, Hollywood gatekeepers said. Be realistic, they told him. It's not going anywhere.

As usual, Arnold paid them no mind, and got to work. He landed his first acting gig in 1970 to play—as fate would have it—Hercules in a low-budget comedy called Hercules in New York, and then burst into the limelight in the 1982 box office hit *Conan the Barbarian*. What followed includes now-iconic films like *Total Recall*, *Predator*, *Terminator*, and *Terminator 2*, and to date, his films have grossed over a billion dollars, making him one of the most successful action movie stars of all time.

Arnold's run for the California governorship was more of the same: no way, no how, impossible, wins handily. Not bad for a starry-eyed Austrian kid nobody believed would, or even should, amount to anything.

This story exemplifies why the gym can give us a lot more than muscle and strength. It can give us more life. Every day we show up and put in the work, it transforms more than our physiques; it transforms our very beings.

So that was the Austrian Oak. What about you? What game do you most want to play? What do you value most? What are your strengths? Who do you most want to become?

Don't sell yourself short when reflecting on these questions. Don't nod along with the reasons why you think you should downsize your dreams. Don't allow the reality of who you currently are snuff out glimmerings of who you could be. Don't skid through life ignoring the music that is inside you.

Recommended Reading
The Magic of Thinking Big by David Schwartz

Do This Now

What's your why for fitness? Why is it a game worth playing? Why do you keep showing up? Reflect on those questions and write your answer down.

Why does that matter? Why is it important to you? How does it benefit you? Reflect on those questions and write your answer down.

Why do those things matter? What do they mean to you? What is special about them? Write your answer down.

Continue this process of asking "why?" until you've written something that *clicks*—that puts a sparkle in your eye and makes you say, "Yes, THAT is really why I do it!" Write this down.

In case you're curious, here's my personal take on this exercise:

What's your why for fitness? Why is it worthwhile? Why do you keep showing up?

To look and feel good and be healthy.

Why does that matter? Why is it important to you? How does it benefit you?

Life is just better when you're happy with what you see in the mirror, when you feel energetic and healthy, and when you don't have to worry about developing disease or dysfunction.

Why does that matter? What does it mean to you? What is special about it?

I want to do a lot of things well in life—personal growth, career, love, friends, etc.—and taking good care of my body will make all of them easier to do. Neglecting my body, however, will make them much harder if not impossible to achieve.

I also want to be a certain type of person. I want to embody the values and ideals I admire, like honesty, honor, diligence, resilience, and independence. As my body is literally the embodiment of my character, taking care of it is closely intertwined with this.

Therefore, when I work out, I'm not just working toward a better-looking body. I'm working toward every single one of my goals and the person I really want to be.

CHAPTER TWO

The Great Art of Sacrifice

"Don't sacrifice who you could be for who you are."
—Dr. Jordan B. Peterson

any years ago, the legendary golfer Gary Player was hitting balls on the range while people looked on in awe.

"Man, I'd give anything to be able to hit a golf ball like you," someone in the gallery called out.

Gary walked over to the man and calmly replied, "No, you wouldn't."

"Yes, I would. I'd give *anything* to hit like that."

"No, you wouldn't," the Hall of Famer repeated. "You wouldn't be willing to do what it takes. You have to rise early in the morning and hit five hundred balls until your hands bleed. Then you stop, tape your hands, and hit five hundred more balls. The next morning, you're out there again with hands so raw you can barely hold your club, but you do it all over again. If you do that through enough years of pain, then you can hit a ball like that."

The man was dumbfounded. Not only was Gary right—he certainly wasn't going to do that—he couldn't believe the pro had to work that hard to make it. He assumed, as many people do, that such an elite performer had ascended to the top of his profession on a balmy updraft of inborn talent and divine providence.

American culture is particularly enamored of this myth. We scorn workaholism and love stories of mysterious prodigies who accomplish great things with effortless grace. We thrill when Matt Damon's character in *Good Will Hunting* scoffs at mathematical proofs that have stumped the brightest minds at MIT—"Do you know how easy this is for me!? This is a fucking joke!" We jeer when captains of industry ascribe their success to sweat, blood, and toil, and we dream of maybe one day stumbling into our own latent superpowers that will put us on the fast track to fame and fortune.

As much as we might want to believe this tale, it's simply not true. While some people come better suited to certain activities than others, decades of research into human performance has made it abundantly clear that both innate talent ("nature") and environmental factors ("nurture") play backseat roles in the development of greatness.

For example, a striking number of legendary artists lived and worked in Renaissance Florence in the fifteenth century, including Leonardo da Vinci, Raphael, Brunelleschi, Michelangelo, Verrocchio, Donatello, and others. Why?

Genes alone can't explain this phenomenon, and neither can environmental considerations. How could so much good DNA accumulate in one place in just a couple of generations, and how were Florence's tumultuous political and economic landscapes conducive to the practice and development of high art? If the nature and nurture theory can't account for this remarkable flowering, what might have caused it?

In Renaissance Florence, it was common for young boys to begin apprenticeships in craft guilds, where they would work under the close supervision of skilled artists. Michelangelo, for instance, began his apprenticeship at age six, starting with stone cutting, followed by sketching and creating frescoes. Leonardo da Vinci didn't get his "big break" until he was forty-six years old, with *The Last Supper*. The genius present in his work wasn't inherited; it was forged through thousands of hours of deep, difficult work.

How many people today marvel at Michelangelo's *David* or Leonardo's *Mona Lisa* and mutter that they'd give anything to be able to sculpt or paint like that? How many people burn for a new body, job, partner, or life and proclaim that they'd do anything to grab ahold of that brass ring? No, they wouldn't. They wouldn't hammer or paint until their hands or eyes bled and then hammer or paint some more. They wouldn't crawl out of bed every day into the cold darkness of dawn to train. They wouldn't burn the midnight oil to become the type of person who *deserves* the better job, partner, or life.

Instead, they actively avoid whatever is difficult and uncomfortable, live according to their feelings and impulses, and decry life's challenges as unfair and people's criticisms as hurtful. They don't want processes and paradigms; they want shortcuts and "hacks." They don't want to plant in the spring and tend in the summer to earn the harvest in the fall; they want to shirk and slack and reap bounties they didn't sow.

In short, they lack the discipline to trade today's pleasure and gratification for tomorrow's security and satisfaction, and if they consider their future prospects at all, they're unrealistically optimistic in their forecasts, envisioning best-case scenarios and not most likely outcomes.

We can sympathize with this plight, though, because let's face it: discipline is hard, maybe one of the hardest skills to learn. All of us are by nature flawed and fickle creatures that aren't wired for scrupulous self-control, but for freewheeling novelty and stimulation. A powerful and primal part of us will blithely repeat what we want to hear instead of telling us how far we still have to go.

How can we outmaneuver and overcome this deep-seated programming?

We can start by evaluating our relationship with *sacrifice*, because while we may say that we want many things in life, if we're not willing to make the right sacrifices to get them, we're just pretending.

Ingmar Bergman was a Swedish director and producer of over sixty films and documentaries and 170 plays, and is widely considered one of the greatest and most influential moviemakers of all time.

"Do you know what moviemaking is?" Bergman asked in a 1964 interview. "Eight hours of hard work each day to get three minutes of film. And during those eight hours there are maybe only ten or twelve minutes, if you're lucky, of real creation. And maybe they don't come. Then you have to gear yourself for another eight hours and pray you're going to get your good ten minutes this time."

For much of Pulitzer Prize winner Toni Morrison's writing career, she worked a day job as an editor at Random House, taught university literature courses, and raised two children as a single mother.

"I am not able to write regularly," she told the *Paris Review* in 1993. "I have never been able to do that—mostly because I always have had a nine-to-five job. I had to write either in between those hours, hurriedly, or spend a lot of weekend and predawn time."

James Joyce estimated that he spent nearly twenty thousand hours writing *Ulysses*. *Twenty thousand hours.* That's nearly seven years working eight hours per day, seven days per week on *one book*—a book that would ultimately become one of the most acclaimed works of fiction ever created.

Frederic Chopin's innovative, nuanced, and technically challenging compositions have established him as one of the greatest composers and pianists of all time, but his creative process was far less harmonious than his masterpieces.

Without foreseeing or seeking it, a melody or tune would come to his mind, and he would then lock himself up in a room for days and begin a desperate, heart-rending quest of trying to get what was in his head down on paper.

He repeated bars hundreds of times, writing and rewriting everything. He once spent six weeks on a single page, only to finish with what he'd first produced. He wept, paced, broke pens, and struggled to find the motivation to get out of bed each day and persevere, and after finally completing a composition, often regretted that what was left wasn't as clearly defined as what he had originally imagined.

While I'm no Bergman, Morrison, Joyce, or Chopin, I can relate to their struggles. I've worked eighty-hour weeks for months on end, I've made mistakes that have cost staggering sums of money, I've weathered organizational and logistical storms that have threatened to put me out of business, and I've poured colossal amounts of time and energy into projects that fell short of expectations or died on the vine.

I've learned, however, that the more of yourself that you're willing to sacrifice to your cause, the less perfect you have to be to succeed. You just have to get enough right, enough of the time.

So, you want a beautiful body, you say?

That's nice, but what are you willing to sacrifice for it? Are you willing to hit the gym every day instead of watching TV? Are you willing to stop eating so much of the "wrong" foods you love so much? Are you willing to give every workout everything you've got?

In other words, do you have the discipline to sacrifice the things you *want* to do for the things you know you *should* do?

If you can't answer these questions with bloodless determination, then you don't really want it, and until you can, you'll never get it. Remember: nothing fails as spectacularly as half measures.

Our culture seems to have forgotten this fundamental law of living. Instead, too many of us believe that life should be predominantly pleasurable, so we constantly search for ways to escape physical and psychological pain. Even our self-help books speak in soft, flattering tones, reassuring us that we're just fine the way we are, and that with enough positive thinking and self-talk, the universe will reward us with abundance and bliss.

This is in stark contrast to times of old, when sacrifice was a sacred act that delighted the gods and earned blessings in return, whether in the form of plentiful harvests, success in war, or personal absolution. In Japan, for example, it was believed that sacrificing a woman at a rushing river would satisfy the spirit who lived there, allowing for the construction of bridges and the safe passage of boats. In the Bible, God sacrificed his only son for the sins of mankind. In Greek myth, Agamemnon killed his own daughter in exchange for a favorable wind on the way to Troy. The great civilizations of Mesoamerica killed people, smashed food, and sank treasure to pay their debts to their gods.

Modernity looks upon such practices and stories as superstitious relics of our barbaric past, and while I wouldn't argue that we should slit a sheep's throat with next January's New Year's resolutions, what do you think might happen if we did? How much more seriously might you take those vows if you had to spill blood over them? And how might society change if everyone else had to do the same?

My point is we have been watching people succeed and fail for thousands of years, and in distilling and codifying our findings and observations, we've learned an important lesson: the people who win make the right sacrifices and the people who lose don't.

That's an unforgiving and unpalatable idea, but also powerful and empowering, because it says that there's no telling what you might be able to do if you're willing to pay the full price. It's also a warning. Life is fraught with peril and suffering, and there are innumerable ways to court chaos and reap the whirlwind. If we want to steer clear of as much catastrophe as possible, then we'd better get serious about making the proper sacrifices now lest we find ourselves forced to make much harder sacrifices later down the line.

What kind of sacrifices should we be making, you might be wondering?

We could start with the obvious: we could stop doing things we know we shouldn't be doing—the things that, if stopped, would immediately make our lives better. You know, things like eating too much sugar or fast food, drinking too much alcohol or doing too many recreational drugs, spending too much time watching TV, playing video games, and using social media, and spending too much money on things we don't really need.

Whatever your list is (and we all have one), take a moment to try to imagine how your life might change over the next year if you were to sacrifice these malignant parts of you.

Now try to imagine what that future might look like if you were to also make the sacrifices of time, attention, and energy necessary to do the things you know you should be doing— eating healthy, exercising regularly, working harder, educating yourself, budgeting and saving money, whatever they might be.

What might happen if you were to do all of that? To what

heights might you rise?

When I self-published a little book called *Bigger Leaner Stronger* in 2012, I had no expectations or grand plans. I had no idea that it would—or even could—go on to sell over three hundred fifty thousand copies (and counting), making it one of the best-selling self-published fitness books of all time, and that I would then go on to write several other best-selling books that would, together, sell over a million copies, and then assemble a team of people and create a multimillion-dollar family of companies including traditional and digital publishing, nutritional supplements, personal coaching, software, and more.

All I knew is writing that first book seemed like something I should do, and so I did it. Each successive development in my career has been guided by the same philosophy and intuition. Once I have committed myself to a desirable outcome, I then try to spend as much time as I can doing things I know will help me get there, and as little time as I can doing things I know will get in the way.

This perspective on sacrifice has abundant support in the scientific literature as well. The classic example is the "Marshmallow Test" that's now synonymous with temptation, willpower, and grit.

This research began in the 1960s at Stanford University, where Walter Mischel taught psychology. Mischel and his graduate students conducted an experiment wherein children were seated in a room and given the choice of their favorite treat, such as a marshmallow, mint, or pretzel, with the option to have one now or two later. The colleague then left the child in the room alone with the goody and told him to speak up if he couldn't wait any longer, and the research team then secretly observed the children to see how they'd handle themselves.

Naturally, many ate the treats straight away, others waited a bit and then gave in, but some managed to hold out until the scientists returned, usually by distracting themselves through singing, playing with their chairs, and other similar activities.

Years later, Mischel and his team followed up with the children and found that those who had successfully waited for the second treat were faring markedly better in life than those who hadn't. They had better SAT scores, education levels, body mass indexes, and personal relationships, and they also rated higher in various life measures including persistence, creativity, foresight, and others.[1]

These studies have since been criticized as inadequate for supporting some of the more sweeping conclusions drawn from them, but I believe the takeaway rings true: the willingness to sacrifice immediate gratification for future rewards is highly correlated with the ability to create a better life.

What most stands in our way of being able to do this, though?

Most people would say they just lack the willpower or self-control, but it's not that simple. While our ability to tap into willpower and exert self-control is influenced by our genetics and upbringing, it's not an immutable element of our biology. We can influence these things greatly through our choices—our mindsets, decisions, and environments.

For example, if we choose to believe that our capacity for self-control is limitless, we'll be far better at regulating our behavior than if we choose to believe it's finite. This has been illustrated in a number of studies, including one conducted by scientists at the University of Maastricht that gave participants a challenge of controlling their facial expressions when shown upsetting video clips.[2]

One group of participants was told that the exercise would be energizing, while the other was told that it would be draining, and after viewing the videos, all participants squeezed a handgrip as hard as they could. The result? The former group performed noticeably better.

Research conducted by scientists at Stanford University echoed these findings, demonstrating that students who believed that tough mental exertion didn't deplete their mental energy didn't show diminished levels of self-control after strenuous experiences and performed much better on their final exams. Students who believed that willpower is a limited resource, however, reported eating more unhealthy food, procrastinating more, and struggling more to prepare for their tests.[3]

Studies also show that we can enhance our self-control by avoiding situations where we have to actively resist temptation.[4]

For instance, if you want to go to a party and drink less, you can choose to sit far from where drinks are being served, or if you're dieting and don't want to eat too much while at a restaurant, you can ask the waiter to not bring the dessert menu or cart, and if you want to focus on studying or working without being distracted by your phone, you can put it on silent and leave it in another room.

While tactics like these are well and good, chances are none of them are particularly striking to you. We instinctively know that if we were truly pushed to the wall, we probably wouldn't choose to die on any of the molehills that we struggle to climb every day.

What is it, then? What's really holding us back?

For many people, it's the fact that it's easy to sacrifice uncertain future rewards for certain immediate ones. Stated differently, it's hard to sacrifice the certain for the uncertain.

That's why we want to savor the junk food today rather than sacrifice it in hopes of a healthier tomorrow, choose the warm embrace of the couch over the austerity of the gym, and consume mindless media instead of meaningful literature.

This tendency to discount future gains is in our nature at least partly because our ancient ancestors had to obsessively chase immediate rewards just to survive—to them, a carrot you had to work years or even decades for was literally unthinkable.

To make matters worse, what do these people do when they finally come face to face with the rotten orchards of their misbegotten desires? Do they reflect on all of their lousy decisions that have made them losers? Rarely. Instead, they whine about how hard and unfair it all is—the rules, competition, and outcomes—and begrudge others their wins.

In his penetrating 2017 memoir-cum-compendium *Principles*, billionaire and hedge fund legend Ray Dalio said the following:

In order to have the best life possible, you must:

1. *know what the best decisions are, and*
2. *have the courage to make them.*

I don't know of any better way to do number one than to analyze the decisions we make every day and ask ourselves what games we're playing and how well we're playing them, and adjusting our investments of time, attention, and effort accordingly.

This approach is uncomfortable, because it requires self-awareness, honesty, knowledge, foresight, and discipline, but we can learn to appreciate and even enjoy the process because of the rewards it provides. In fact, if we can stay the course, this almost happens automatically, because regardless of how foreign it might feel at first, the more we do something, the more we come to like it and want to continue doing it.

Evidence of this can be found in seminal research conducted by Robert B. Zajonc and published in 1968 that demonstrated that "mere exposure" to an arbitrary stimulus generates "mild affection" for it.[5] This holds true with nonsense phrases, human faces, Chinese ideographs, and other visual stimuli, as well as sounds, tastes, ideas, and social interactions of all kinds.

Marketers and politicians have known the power of repeated exposure for at least as long, and it explains why they spend vast sums of money to repeat simple slogans, jingles, and messages again and again. They know that the more you see and hear their statements, the more familiar and acceptable their products, services, and ideas will become to you.

This is why GEICO spends over a billion dollars per year creating and propagating silly but memorable commercials that have little to do with the benefits of insurance, and why political parties are so adamant that their members stay "on message," repeating the same talking points as publicly and frequently as possible.

What this means for our discussion is that while sacrificing immediate gratification may be difficult and awkward at first, the more we do it, the easier it becomes. It's just a habit that we can establish like any other, and as such, it can take time to settle into. Specifically, studies show that new habits can take anywhere from a couple weeks to a couple months or longer to stick, with most people needing about sixty-six days to internalize new behavior patterns.[6]

The key, then, is making it through the first two months, and there are several psychological "tricks" we can employ to increase our chances of success.

One way to deal effectively with temptation to act against your long-term interests is to view the choice as giving up the long-term reward for whatever you find immediately enticing. Take a moment to imagine what it would feel like to enjoy the ultimate payoff, and bask in the fruits of your self-control. Then ask if you're willing to throw all that away for the fleeting pleasure of whatever form of instant gratification you're faced with. How does that trade make you feel? Is it worth it?

Let's say you're on a quest to lose fifteen pounds, and are

staring down a plate of your favorite confections. Close your eyes for a minute, and imagine having reached your goal weight. Feel how your clothes fit, picture how your new body looks in the mirror, and hear the compliments from friends and loved ones. Now open your eyes, and ask yourself: Do you want that or the temporary delight of a dollop of sugar and fat? Chances are the desserts will look a lot less appetizing.

This line of thinking not only helps us negotiate moments of temptation—it also highlights the fact that every transgression has real-world ramifications. The penalties are rarely obvious or immediately felt, however. They accrue insidiously, like a growing thunderhead, until a predestined moment in the future, when they will unleash their pent-up fury upon us. Here is the smoker who receives the soul-shattering diagnosis, the glutton whose heart gives out, the cheater wracked by guilt, and the ne'er-do-well devoid of self-respect.

Similarly, every time we act nobly, tangible benefits may not materialize before our eyes, but they too accrue, inevitably manifesting in all manner of ways. There is always an immediate payoff in doing right by you, however, and it's the emotional reward of feeling good about your choices.

Sophisticated marketers exploit this psychology with a technique known as laddering, which boils down to persuading people that buying a product or service will immediately make them feel the way they would like to feel.

For example, to sell faster processing speed on a mobile device, it might go like this: a faster processor means less waiting, less waiting means accomplishing more, and accomplishing more means feeling more in charge and powerful. Advertisements, then, would be aimed at convincing you that the minute you buy the faster phone, you'll enjoy the immediate, certain, and emotional reward of feeling commanding.

We can use this psychological tactic to our advantage,

because while the concrete rewards of making good decisions may be delayed and uncertain, the emotional ones are always instantaneous and assured. By focusing on the latter, we can gain considerable power over our behavior. We can consider how it will *feel* to smoke or drink less or stick to our diet or exercise routine instead of how it will benefit our physiology; how it will *feel* to see our savings rise or debts fall, instead of how it will impact our net worth or financial resilience; how it will *feel* to spend less time on social media or watching TV, instead of how it will free up time for other valuable activities.

Yet another method of short-circuiting a momentary desire is putting whatever is tempting you out of sight. This works because not being able to see the immediate reward makes it less exciting to our primitive selves, and thus easier to reject.

For example, one study conducted by scientists at the University of Illinois found that office workers who kept a jar of candy inside their desk drawer consumed considerably less than those who kept it on their desks.[7] It's not harder to reach into a drawer than across a desk, but putting the goodies out of sight helped put them out of mind.

Similar results were seen in another study conducted by scientists at the University of Cambridge.[8] In this case, participants were told they were part of a "relaxation and personality" exercise, and were placed in a room with a few magazines and a bowl of candy for ten minutes.

For one group of participants, the bowl was very close— about twenty centimeters away—and for the other, a little farther—about seventy centimeters away. Researchers found that the people who were seventy centimeters away from the candy ate, on average, 40 percent less than those who were closer.

In another variation of the same study, the participants were exposed to the same situation and then given a memorization problem to solve (to induce mental fatigue), and then re-exposed to the conditions. The outcome was the same, indicating that the reduction in candy eating wasn't a matter of cognitive effort required to reach for it, but mere proximity.[8]

You can also institute a mandatory ten-minute wait before allowing yourself to indulge in an undesirable activity. This may not seem like much time, but research conducted by scientists at Princeton University shows that it can make a big difference in how you perceive the situation.[9]

In short, the part of you that wants immediate gratification wants it *now*, and if you resolve to delay for just ten minutes, it no longer sees an instant reward but a future one, allowing you to cool off and make the wiser choice.

So in the case of the showdown with desserts discussed earlier, if ten minutes of waiting (and visualizing the long-term reward at stake) isn't enough to squash the desire to indulge, then allow yourself to, but not before.

Flip this around, and you have a powerful strategy for fighting procrastination. Decide to do whatever you're dreading for just ten minutes, and once they're up, allow yourself to stop. Chances are you'll want to keep going!

Yet another highly effective strategy for training your willpower is called "precommitment," which entails taking action now to strengthen your position and commitment to a behavior and ward off any underhanded attempts at self-sabotage.

Much like how Ulysses instructed his men to lash him to the mast of their ship to ensure he didn't fall prey to the beautiful songs of the sea Sirens, you too can create systems to protect you from your lower self. With the right precommitment strategies, you can put safeguards in place that make it nearly impossible to fail.

For instance, if you have trouble with procrastinating on the internet instead of working, you can download a program called Cold Turkey (www.getcoldturkey.com) that allows you to block specific websites and applications or turn your internet off altogether for a set period of time.

If sticking to a diet is your struggle, you could precommit by throwing out all tempting junk foods in the house and not rebuying them, preparing healthy lunches to bring to work every day, and putting money on the line on a website like www.dietbet.com.

If you want to precommit to exercising regularly, you could pay for an annual membership at your gym instead of going month-to-month, or sign up for an online coaching service.

Another tool that has helped many thousands of people precommit successfully to all kinds of goals is the website www.stickk.com.

Stickk allows you to set a goal and time frame, wager money, and decide what happens with it if you fail. (It could go to a charity, for example, or even an organization you don't like, which can be a stronger incentive.) You can also designate a "referee" who will monitor your progress and confirm the truthfulness of your reports, and invite supporters to cheer you on.

So, remember this: every moment of every day, we're making sacrifices of time, energy, and attention. Are they the right sacrifices, though? The sacrifices that accrue rewards instead of retributions? The sacrifices needed to make things better?

Are we moving past listlessness and cravings for ease and comfort and developing the discipline to focus our minds and efforts on future benefits, or are we still acting like children, succumbing to our shortsighted primitive instincts? Are we making the right bargains with the future, or selling ourselves short?

These are some of the fundamental questions that we must

reflect on regularly, and the body and life that we ultimately create will be our answers.

I interviewed author and former Navy SEAL Mark Divine on my podcast a couple of years ago, and he shared his experience of the infamous "Hell Week" that recruits have to survive (literally) to advance to the next round of training and selection.

This ordeal was designed with one purpose in mind—to break people in body, mind, and spirit—and after the first few days, Mark feared he wasn't going to make it. Nothing could have prepared him for the nightmarish conditions, which included extreme sleep deprivation, relentless running, rowing, and rolling in the frigid shores of Coronado, California, and merciless hectoring from drill instructors whose job was to cull the weak from the herd.

All he had to do, his superiors reminded him every hour, was ring a bell on the beach, and all the agony would end. Salvation was always at hand. And so Mark had to make a decision as he sat in the pounding surf, shivering and shaking violently: How badly did he want to become an "operator"? What was it worth to him?

"I decided that I would keep going until I died," he told me in the interview. "And then it got a whole lot easier. Am I dead yet? No? Then I can keep going."

Many people think that finding answers to the right questions is the "secret" to setting and achieving goals. They're wrong. That's the easy part. The secret is facing the answers.

How much pain are you willing to take? What are you willing to sacrifice? How far are you willing to go?

And know this: It's always going to be harder than you

think. It's always going to take more time, effort, and energy than you want to give. You're always going to face more seductions to stray than you think you can resist. And you're always going to suffer more setbacks and shocks than you feel is fair.

If you can clear those hurdles, though, then there's quite literally nothing that can stop you except death itself.

Recommended Reading

12 Rules for Life by Jordan B. Peterson

Do This Now

The ability to sacrifice the present for the future is a skill you can practice. Like any other skill, the more you practice it, the better you get, and the better you get, the better you can do it in any area of your life.

To start this process of improvement, take the following seven-day challenge. Each day will involve sacrificing something you probably find desirable and pleasurable for something that may not tickle the neurons, but will certainly toughen them.

DAY ONE
Take a Cold Shower

Research shows that cold showers aren't going to help you

lose fat faster, increase your testosterone levels, boost your post-workout recovery, strengthen your immune system, or give you prettier skin or hair, but they most definitely will do this:[10]

They'll make you really uncomfortable.

And that's why they're a great way to kick off the challenge. Specifically, here's what you need to do:

1. Set your shower to its coldest setting, and let it run for a couple of minutes (ensuring the water is as cold as possible).
2. Go in head-first. Don't start with your toes and slowly work up your body.
3. Spend at least three minutes under the water, rotating every minute or so, ensuring your entire body is wet.
4. Optional: Reward yourself with hot water after the cold is complete. Or not, if you're willing to sacrifice that too. :-)

DAY TWO
No Caffeine or Refined Sugar

Caffeine and sugar are two molecules that make the world go 'round, and that's why you're going to give them up for a day.

And that means giving them up *completely* for twenty-four hours—not a single ounce of coffee or caffeinated tea or gram of refined sugar in any of its sneaky forms, like sucrose, high-fructose corn syrup (HFCS), evaporated cane juice, or dextrose.

DAY THREE
Digital Detox

The entire idea of "detoxing" the body through cleanses, teas, and supplements is outright quackery, but a regular "digital detox" through tech-free time can be well worth it.

For instance, studies show that dialing down our use of devices can improve our sleep, make us less narcissistic, improve our mental health, and help us maintain a healthy relationship with our screened devices.[11]

The *how* here is simple: absolutely no tech for twenty-four hours—no smartphone, tablet, computer, television, or anything else with a screen.

This is easiest to do on a weekend day, of course, so feel free to start this seven-day challenge on a Thursday or Friday (or swap this day with another so it falls on a Saturday or Sunday).

DAY FOUR
No Highly Processed Foods

You don't have to obsessively eat "clean" foods to be lean, muscular, and healthy. So long as you're getting the majority of your calories from nutritious, relatively unprocessed foods, you're doing it right.

Unfortunately, however, most people don't do that, and eat far too much low-quality, nutritionally bankrupt food instead. That's why today's challenge is to eat well for twenty-four hours.

Practically speaking, that means sticking to simple, "healthy" foods like fruits, vegetables, whole grains, nuts, seeds, legumes, and lean proteins—foods that you have to prepare and cook yourself.

If you want to make this as easy as possible, you can follow one of the "clean eating" meal plans provided in the bonus material at www.workoutmotivationbook.com/bonus.

DAY FIVE
One Hour of Cardiovascular Exercise

Cardiovascular exercise can benefit your health in many ways, even if you already do regular resistance training.

It can also be extremely uncomfortable, and so on this day, you're going to do an hour of it.

What kind you do is up to you, but here's the rub: it has to be hard. So if you're very out of shape, maybe it's an hour of walking, and if you're very fit, it may be an hour of vigorous jogging.

Happy trails!

DAY SIX
Wake Up Earlier

If you read a bunch of personal transformation stories on websites like Quora or Reddit, you'll quickly notice that many of them involve waking up earlier.

Why?

A number of reasons:

1. It allows you to trade "dead time," where you're passive and biding your time, for "alive time," where you're engaged with life and doing something meaningful. By going to bed and waking up earlier, you'll naturally

spend less time doing things you feel you should do less of, and gain more time for things that are important to you, like exercise, reading, goal setting, meditating, working, or journaling.

2. It allows you to experience the joy of quietude. The early morning hours are peaceful and calm, with no kids or babies squawking, cars rumbling, or devices buzzing.

3. It allows you to appreciate the beauty of the sunrise. Every day, nature greets us with a stunning vista of blues, reds, oranges, and purples. Missing it is a shame.

4. It allows you to be more productive.Even if you're not a "morning person," you can become one, and when you do, you'll get more productive work done every day. Period. By doing your most important work first thing, before the distractions of the office and life kick into high gear, you might be surprised at just how much progress you can make on your most meaningful projects.

So, on this wonderful day, wake up ninety minutes earlier than usual (this should be easier than an hour or even thirty minutes earlier due to your body's natural sleep rhythms), and then use that time wisely!

A few tips for succeeding in this challenge:

1. Go to bed two hours earlier than usual.
   The idea here isn't to sleep–deprive yourself for a day, but to experience the benefits of both waking up early and being well rested.

2. Put your alarm clock far from your bed.
   You snooze, and you lose. By forcing yourself to get up to turn off the alarm, you'll be up.

3.   Leave the bedroom after turning off your alarm.
     Whatever you do, don't let your brain trick you into going back to bed. Force yourself out of the bedroom.

DAY SEVEN
Leaving the Shallows

Attention spans may not be dwindling as quickly as many people believe, but there's no question that we often have an overwhelming number of internal and external stimuli vying for our attention.[12]

This has heightened many people's desire for distraction, and research shows that the more our brains become accustomed to on-demand diversion, the harder it is to sweep aside and concentrate.[13]

To quote Cal Newport in his stimulating 2016 book *Deep Work*:

> . . . *the use of a distracting service does not, by itself, reduce your brain's ability to focus. It's instead the constant switching from low-stimuli/high-value activities to high-stimuli/low-value activities, at the slightest hint of boredom or cognitive challenge, that teaches your mind to never tolerate an absence of novelty.*

It's also self-evident that our ability to get on in the world is going to depend greatly upon our ability to manage our attention. Who we become, what we learn and accomplish, and who's with us in the end will ensue directly from the things we pay the most attention to day after day and year after year.

This is why Newport says that we should train our ability to concentrate intensely and overcome our desire for distraction, and that's the purpose of this challenge, which will have you do a bit of "productive meditation."

Specifically, I want you to take a period in which you're occupied physically but not mentally—like walking, jogging, or showering—and focus your attention on a single, well-defined issue, opportunity, or problem.

This could be a professional concern, like outlining an article, crafting a marketing plan, or sharpening a business strategy; a personal affair, like having a difficult talk with a partner, creating a new diet or exercise program, or figuring out how to save more money; or anything else that would improve your life if completed or resolved.

Whatever you've chosen, your goal in this challenge is to concentrate solely on it for at least fifteen minutes (up to as long as you can) and bring it closer to completion or resolution.

You're probably going to struggle at first—your attention is probably going to dart, wander, and stall—and that's okay. When this happens, gently remind yourself that you can think about whatever comes to mind later, bring your attention back to the issue at hand, and carry on.

Look out for what Newport calls "looping," as well, where your mind loops over and over again on something you've already considered or realized instead of diving deeper and generating new ideas.

When you notice this happening, acknowledge that you seem to be in a loop, and then focus on the next (new) step in the process.

CHAPTER THREE

The Trouble with Waiting for Perfect

"The Way of the Samurai is in desperateness. Ten men or more cannot kill such a man. Common sense will not accomplish great things. Simply become insane and desperate."
—Lord Naoshige

Think of something in your life you'd like to improve. Just one thing you'd like to add, change, or remove. Got it? Good.

Now think of a few ideas of how you might move that needle.

If you'd like to have more money, what are a few ways you could make some extra cash? Get creative!

Want some help?

- Sell your skills on sites like TaskRabbit and Thumbtack.
- Learn to code web pages, and offer your services to local businesses.

- Rent out a room in your house.
- Teach stuff you know on sites like Udemy or Skillshare.
- Become a "field agent" and help businesses do market research.
- Make cool stuff and sell it on Etsy.
- Deliver people's groceries with Instacart.
- Walk people's dogs.

Or maybe you'd like to lose some fat and build some muscle? Okay, let's brainstorm.

- Make a proper meal plan.
- Eat no fast food for a month.
- Learn how to use portion control to your advantage.
- Stop buying foods you tend to overeat.
- Lift heavy weights a few times per week.
- Do a few high-intensity interval cardio workouts per week.
- Go for a long walk every morning.

Or maybe you'd like to save more money, read more books, or learn a new skill? Go ahead and make the list. I'll wait.

My point is no matter what you'd like to change in your life, it's easy to compile a lengthy list of feasible ways to do it.

The real question is why you're not doing any of those things. Why haven't you started? What are you waiting for? For the perfect moment? The perfect mood? The perfect day? For all your imaginary ducks to get in a row?

Let's face it: conditions will never be just right. Perfect is just an excuse that we use to stay comfortable and ensconced in the status quo.

When someone says they're going to do that one thing "one of these days," we all know the truth—if they haven't carved out the time and energy already, they probably never will. They'll keep dreaming instead of doing, until they eventually can't even bring themselves to dream anymore.

Napoleon Bonaparte once said, "Sometimes death only comes from a lack of energy." Well, the surest way to suffer from a lack of energy is having a lack of ideas and challenges, from shouldering less burden than we can carry. In this way, waiting for perfect is a perfect way to die a little every day.

The only choice, then, is to stop telling ourselves that we need things to be "just right" before we can start doing the thing. It'll never happen. Start now, and figure it out as you go. You can sit around and wait for the inspiration to run a marathon, or you can get up right now and go for a ten-minute jog. You can wait for the stars to align before starting that side hustle, or you can skip Netflix tonight and start reading on where to begin.

If you do this—if you can cast aside your fears, doubts, and anxieties and just get into action instead—you'll begin a process far more profound than you probably realize. You'll find that the more you do, the more your attitudes and feelings will shift. Limiting opinions and rationalizations that were once dear to you will crumble and fade away. Behaviors that first felt alien and formidable will become familiar and routine.

In time, you'll become the rare type of person who is actually doing the thing.

Elon Musk personifies this notion of acting boldly in the face of highly incomplete and imperfect information and circumstances. Take the origin story of SpaceX, for instance, a company whose stated purpose is to revolutionize space travel and help humans colonize Mars by the end of this century.

"For a long time," Elon told hedge fund giant Ray Dalio, "I've thought that it's inevitable that something bad is going to happen on a planetary scale—a plague, a meteor—that will require humanity to start over somewhere else, like Mars. One day I went to the NASA website to see what progress they were making on their Mars program, and I realized that they weren't even thinking about going there anytime soon.

"I had gotten $180 million when my partners and I sold PayPal," he continued, "and it occurred to me that if I spent $90 million and used it to acquire some ICBMs from the former USSR and sent one to Mars, I could inspire the exploration of Mars."

When Ray asked him about his background in rocketry, he told him he didn't have one. "I just started reading books," he said.

And in fact, this venturesome spirit is the only way to "be like Elon." Many people mistakenly believe—or want to believe—that you first have to change your mind before you can change anything else. That you have to find your balance before you can run.

Research conducted by scientists at the University of Wisconsin–Milwaukee suggests that this is exactly backward— that the surest way to change attitude is to change behavior, and that the reverse rarely works.[1] You might think you need to wait for balance before running, but it's in the running itself that you usually find it.

The reason for this is we derive our attitudes from how we behave, and figure out who we are by watching what we do. Therefore, when we act in a way that's inconsistent with our current attitudes and beliefs, regardless of why, we will generally adjust the subjective to match the objective, not the other way around. In other words, we'll adjust our mental models to make sense of our behaviors, even if they're deceptive, disgraceful, or downright dreadful.

In this way, every single thing we do every day molds and determines our self-definition to one degree or another. We can think all the best thoughts with all the right intentions, but unless our actions embody them, we'll reinterpret it all to rationalize our shortcomings. And the more intelligent we are, the better we're going to be at making excuses, creating a powerful, self-reinforcing, vicious cycle of degradation.

Many people say many of the obstacles we face in life are of our own creation—the limitations, restrictions, and criticisms we impose on ourselves. This is probably true. It's also true, though, that the only way to clear these hurdles is through our willingness and ability to take action regardless of how we feel at first blush, and then to resist temptations to lose psychological ground by acting otherwise. How well we can do that and that alone will ultimately determine our fate more than anything else.

In *Alice in Wonderland*, the Red Queen says that in her race, you have to run as fast as you can just to stay in place, and twice as fast as that to go anywhere. This is a perfect metaphor for life. You have to hustle just to pass muster, and work twice as hard as that to gain ground.

I opened this chapter with a quote from the legendary Samurai general Lord Naoshige, whose story and sayings are found in the timeless book *Hagakure*:

> *The Way of the Samurai is in desperateness. Ten men or more cannot kill such a man. Common sense will not accomplish great things. Simply become insane and desperate.*

I believe his words are just as true today as they were four hundred years ago, if not more so.

Modern "common sense" says you shouldn't work too hard. That you shouldn't become too obsessed with a goal. That you should release yourself from the burdens of desire and pursuit and just be thankful for what you have.

These philosophies are quickly embraced by the more

"well-adjusted" members of society. To these people, you must be "insane" if you're going to make it. Insane to work twice as hard as everyone you know, insane to wake up at the crack of dawn to get in your workouts, insane to pursue goals they don't understand and take risks they can't imagine.

Many of these people will delight in telling you as much too. In fact, they'll have so much advice that if you were to scribble it all down on pieces of paper, you'd singlehandedly decimate entire swaths of the world's forests. Always keep your eyes and ears open, but don't let their moonshine move you off target.

"You shouldn't do that," they'll say, wheeling out a litany of reasons why it's not going to work out, why you should squander your life like they do, and why you'll regret it if you keep going.

And then you'll say, "Screw it. I'm doing it anyway."

"Screw it. I'm going to count my calories and lose those twenty pounds."

"Screw it. I'm going to follow that workout program for a couple months."

"Screw it. I'm going to clean up my diet."

You'll probably be afraid too. Anxious. Uncertain. All that is normal. Remember the first time you rode a bike? This is no different. All you have to do is shrug, mutter "Who gives a shit?" and get to work. You put in work, and you get better. You get better, and you gain confidence. You gain confidence, and you want to do more good work. It's a virtuous cycle.

The hobgoblins of fear and doubt will always hop around in your mind, sometimes more noisily than others, and that's okay. Some of it is even good; it keeps you moving, doing, working. It reminds you that the best way out is the way through.

I dance with these bogeymen every time I start in on something new. "What if everyone hates it?" one might chirp. "What if you can't pull it off?" another might chime in. "What if it blows up in your face?" another might squawk.

This is how I know I'm on the right path, that I've identified a challenge worth pursuing. If I'm not facing a new insecurity, then I know I'm not stretching far enough.

"Insane" isn't enough, according to Lord Naoshige. You have to be *desperate* too. What's desperation? Napoleon Bonaparte said that "death is nothing, but to live defeated is to die every day." *That's* desperation. It's the feeling that you must not be beaten. That everything is on the line. That only an all-in commitment is appropriate, and that the only excuse for failure is simply a failure of will.

"Until one is committed, there is hesitancy, the chance to draw back, always ineffectiveness," said the mountaineer and writer W.H. Murray. "Concerning all acts of initiative (and creation), there is one elementary truth, the ignorance of which kills countless ideas and splendid plans: that the moment one definitely commits oneself, then Providence moves too. All sorts of things occur to help one that would never otherwise have occurred. A whole stream of events issues from the decision, raising in one's favour all manner of unforeseen incidents and meetings and material assistance, which no man could have dreamt would have come his way. I have learned a deep respect for one of Goethe's couplets: Whatever you can do, or dream you can, begin it. Boldness has genius, power, and magic in it!"

Years ago, I would have dismissed this as mysticism or myth. I've now experienced it enough to be fully convinced of the phenomenon. The more determined I am to see something through to a full and proper conclusion, the more it goes right, and often in ways that you can only chalk up to serendipity— unlikely opportunities, timely coincidences, and lucky lifelines.

For whatever reason, intention seems to be a force multiplier of sorts, and work done with resolve seems to outpace work done with a wavering mind.

I can clearly remember the watershed moment when I

decided to go for broke as a fitness author and entrepreneur, despite initially rejecting the idea.

I balked at first, because as much as I love health, fitness, and helping others, I really don't love the health and fitness community and culture, which is overrun with liars, narcissists, and neurotics. Not exactly my scene.

Furthermore, I only had one self-published book that was achieving moderate success, but no real following, friends, or even allies in the space, which is notoriously competitive and unreceptive to upstarts trying to make their bones.

I considered all of this carefully, but chose to make the leap of faith anyway, for three reasons:

1. I was merely a competent writer, but that was enough to produce books and articles considerably better than most others in the space, and I knew I could vastly improve in this regard and gain even more ground.
2. Many of the people who would be my competitors were lazy, complacent, and disorganized by my standards, and I was certain I could outwork and out-marshal them by an order of magnitude.
3. Many of these people were also poor businesspeople and marketers, and I was fairly certain I could outmaneuver them in those areas as well.

My deliberation ended with a hard-line decision:

I was going to do whatever it took to capitalize on this opportunity and make a splash in the fitness space.

And it has been a rocket ride.

Sure, my team and I have made plenty of missteps and suffered some painful blows, but we've also made enough astute judgments and strategic moves, spent enough time at the coalface, and gotten enough lucky breaks to establish a multifaceted, multimillion-dollar conglomerate of companies.

So, that's me. What about you. What would you like to make happen?

Well, what are you waiting for? The clock is ticking. To quote from the *Hagakure* again:

> *Death seems a long way off. Is this not shallow thinking? It is worthless and is only a joke within a dream [. . .] Insofar as death is always at one's door, one should make sufficient effort and act quickly.*

It's time to decide. Are you insane and desperate enough to do what needs to be done?

Recommended Reading
The Subtle Art of Not Giving a F*ck by Mark Manson

Do This Now

In his blockbuster book on productivity, *Getting Things Done*, David Allen shares a simple system for capturing what has our attention, clarifying what each item means and what to do about it, and organizing and optimizing our efforts.

A major component of his "GTD" philosophy is breaking complex, overwhelming tasks into small, manageable tasks, and then starting on the first one.

One of the exercises Allen recommends is taking the things that have our attention (concerns, worries, problems, issues, tensions) and translating them into achievable outcomes (projects), to be executed with concrete next actions.

Let's get a taste of this.

Write down the three things that are most on your mind these days. Don't exclude something because you think it might be irrelevant. If it's on your mind a lot, there's a reason, so it's probably a good idea to tackle it now rather than later.

"Many of us hold ourselves back from imagining a desired outcome unless someone can show us how to get there," Allen says in the book. "Unfortunately, that's backward in terms of how our minds work to generate and recognize solutions and methods. [. . .] "There is a simple but profound principle that emerges from understanding the way your perceptive filters work: you won't see how to do it until you see yourself doing it.

"You often need to make it up in your mind before you can make it happen in your life."

Next, then, visualize and write down the exact outcomes you desire for these affairs.

For instance, how might your body look and feel if your diet and exercise regimens were to work out? How might that work project look if it were done well? How might your relationship with your significant other feel if the conversation you need to have went well?

Whatever your three "to-be-addressed" things are, envision what success will ultimately look like for each, and write it all down.

Now it's time to brainstorm ideas as to how you might move toward those desired outcomes.

What could you do to go from where you are to at least slightly closer to where you want to be?

Don't judge, challenge, or evaluate these ideas yet—just let them flow and write them down. Go for quantity here, not quality.

Next, let's drill down to "next actions," which Allen defines as physical, visible activities that would be required to move the situation toward closure.

For example, throwing away all the junk food you tend to overeat so you can better stick to your diet, calling three local gyms to get information on their classes, and buying an inexpensive upright bike so you can easily do cardio at home would all be good next actions.

Formulate one single next action for each of your three concerns that would, once completed, bring you one step closer to the desired results, and write them down.

Also, if any of these projects (as Allen would call them) have multiple components or aspects, feel free to generate a single next action for each of the moving parts.

Allow me to provide a personal example of this exercise.

1. *Write down the three things that are most on your mind these days.*
   A. Completing the rather long lineup of important work projects on my plate, including finishing and launching this book, updating *Bigger Leaner Stronger* and *Thinner Leaner Stronge*r, closing my first traditional book deal, getting more publicity, launching my first four Muscle for Life digital courses, and scaling up Legion's advertising.
   B. Improving the quality of my sleep, as it has gotten worse over the last few years. (I wake up at least once or twice most nights, whereas I used to sleep straight through.)
   C. Improving the quality of the time I spend with my wife and kids, as I feel I'm often not making it maximally rewarding to all.

2. *Visualize and write down the exact outcomes you desire for these affairs.*

   A. The timely and successful completion of the projects that have the greatest potential to impact the growth of my companies and brands.

   B. Regular uninterrupted and restful sleep.

   C. Regular highly positive and satisfying experiences with my family that foster joy, love, and intimacy for all four of us.

3. *Now it's time to brainstorm ideas as to how you might move toward those desired outcomes.*

   A. Clearly prioritize projects based on estimated time, difficulty, and payoff; create a comprehensive action plan for the highest-priority project; track and assess everything I'm currently spending time on to see what can be delegated or eliminated to free up time for more important things; roadmap the action plan into my work schedule to determine how quickly it could get done; and repeat the planning and scheduling process for any other tasks and projects that must be done concurrently.

   B. I've already tried quite a few things to improve my sleep with spotty results, but I'm homing in on the problem, which is twofold:

      a.) I'm a lighter sleeper than I was years ago.

      b.) I'm more sensitive to caffeine as well.

   Therefore, I've stopped playing white noise when I sleep, and limited my caffeine intake to about 120 milligrams on the weekdays and none on the weekends, and this has helped tremendously.

The problem isn't 100 percent resolved, though, and completely eliminating caffeine for a week didn't make any difference. So, next, I could create a relaxing pre-bed routine that could include things proven to help activate the parasympathetic nervous system, like taking a hot bath, doing a breathing exercise, listening to soothing music, and so on.

C. I can plan specific activities for family time that everyone will enjoy, so we're not scrambling last-minute to come up with things to do.

4. *Next, let's drill down to "next actions," which Allen defines as physical, visible activities that would be required to move the situation toward closure.*

A. Assess the projects I have in front of me in terms of estimated time, difficulty, and payoff to determine which ones should be tackled first.

B. Create a relatively short pre-bed routine for relaxing that I can do every night.

C. Brainstorm family activities with my wife, Sarah.

SETTING THE GOALS

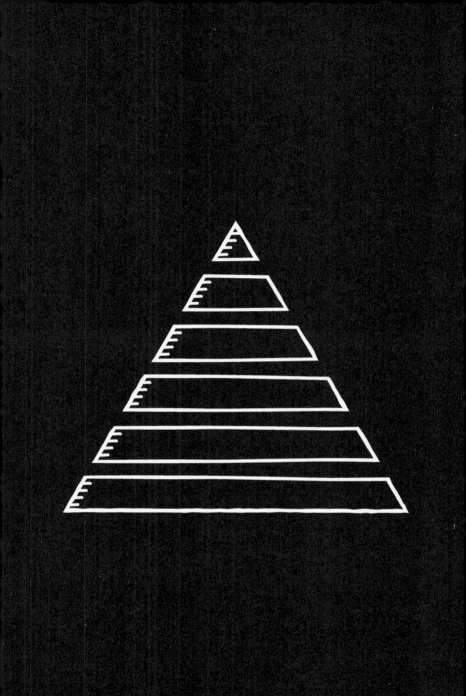

CHAPTER FOUR

The Greatest Common Denominator of Greatness

"If you want to live a happy life, tie it to a goal, not to people or things."
—Albert Einstein

very great story of adventure has a point of no return, where there's no turning back. If the hero is to carry on, he must abandon life as he knew it and give himself fully to what lies ahead.

Dorothy lives in a one-room house on a sun-scorched, treeless prairie with her dreary aunt and uncle. Her only source of happiness is her dog, Toto. A twister rips through the plains one day and carries her to the lush Munchkin Country in the Land of Oz. To return home, she must venture to the Emerald City and meet the mysterious Wizard of Oz.

Rome breaches its land treaty with Carthage, and Hannibal retaliates by laying siege to the Roman protectorate of Saguntum. Rome demands justice from Carthage, but instead war is declared, and the Second Punic War begins. Hannibal's numbers are far inferior to the mighty Roman Empire, but his military brilliance and daring bring it to the edge of collapse.

Siddhārtha Gautama is born into a royal Hindu family, destined to enjoy a life of privilege and luxury. One day, he leaves his palace to meet his subjects, and witnesses human suffering and the decay of old age for the first time. His utopia-shattering experience motivates further trips beyond the palace walls. Eventually, his conscience drives him to escape his sheltered, princely life and unite his people in pursuit of a spiritual solution to misery.

Each of these people had goals: the goal of returning home, the goal of vanquishing a mighty oppressor, the goal of rejuvenating an entire people. Goals fuel action, because goals give us purpose, and purpose is what inspires us, lights us up, and floats our boats. We can only become fully engaged in life when we feel that we are doing something that really matters. Only in purpose can we find the strength to cross our own Rubicons and march toward a better future.

This is why the search for purpose and meaning is one of the most powerful and lasting themes in every culture since the dawn of time.

You'll find it in Homer's *Odyssey*, and it has inspired some of the greatest spiritual figures in history: Jesus, Buddha, Moses, Muhammad, and countless other venerated saints and prophets. You'll even find this search in modern culture, in movies like *Indiana Jones and the Last Crusade*, which retells the story of Perceval's search for the Holy Grail through the daring character of Indiana Jones, and the famous *Star Wars* trilogy, in which Luke Skywalker confronts his deepest fears by overcoming Darth

Vader and the Empire. It's no coincidence that these movies, telling the legendary tale of the search for significance and the struggle of good versus evil, are among the most successful of all time.

Goals are the milestones you create for your journey. They determine how far you will go, and how you will know when you've accomplished something worthwhile. They are vessels into which you pour your curiosity, imagination, passion, and sweat, and they fill you with drive, enthusiasm, and joy.

For goals to do all this, though, they must be handled skillfully, because when you say that you're going to accomplish something, you're placing the core of your very being on the line. Your self-identity, self-respect, and self-efficacy are at stake, and failing to do what you set out to do can cut right to the bone.

This is why goals are to be respected. Feared, even. Trifle with them at your own risk, because they can break you— they can split you open and lay bare your every weakness and insecurity. Some people's spirits just never recover from their disastrous encounters with big goals. If you don't feel at least a twinge of sobriety or humility before starting in on a meaningful aim, you're probably going to fail. Don't pull up the anchor just yet.

And so a discussion about goal setting and attainment is in order, because if you can get this right, you can greatly increase your chances of long-term success and satisfaction inside and outside the gym.

Recommended Reading
Hard Goals by Mark Murphy

Do This Now

Who do you know who has poured their curiosity, imagination, passion, and sweat into their goals and made them a reality? What did they do that you admire? Write your answers down.

If you truly don't know anybody that fits this criterion, then who have you learned about who does? What did they do?

If the person (or persons) you wrote is someone you know, have you told them that you admire how they've handled themselves? That they inspire you to reach for your own goals?

If not, do that now! It'll make their day!

In case you'd like to know my take on this, for me, it's my father, who's a successful entrepreneur, philanthropist, and all-around mensch, as well as people I've read about whose stories have inspired me and shaped my ideas, attitudes, and behaviors, including Theodore Roosevelt, Alexander the Great, Elon Musk, John D. Rockefeller, and Leonardo da Vinci.

I admire these people for a number of reasons, and have learned and benefited a lot from them. I don't want to bore you with all of the details, but here's the flavor:

- I admire my dad's compassion and generosity, and have used this to help me better navigate ticklish situations I've faced.
- I admire Teddy Roosevelt's wisdom, courage, and zeal, and have modeled some of my personal standards and ambitions on his attitudes and behaviors.
- I admire Alexander the Great's and Elon Musk's force of will, and have drawn encouragement from their lives to aspire to do and be more than I think I can.
- I admire John D. Rockefeller's tenacity and single-mindedness, and I have applied a number of the lessons

I've gleaned from his story to improve my work and business.

- I admire Leonardo da Vinci's curiosity and integrity, and have found in him inspiration to march to the beat of my own drum despite what other people might think.

CHAPTER FIVE

The Wrong Way and Right Way to Set Goals

*"Even if you fail at your ambitious thing, it's very hard
to fail completely. That's the thing
people don't get."*
—Larry Page

I f you're like most people, you start goal setting by asking a simple question: "What do I want?"

This is a fine place to begin, but if you don't answer this question in a very specific way, your chances of actually achieving anything worthwhile plummet.

The first step in processing your rough-hewn desires into functional goals is getting specific, because while vague goals may seem more motivating at first, they quickly lose their steam if left that way.

This has been demonstrated in a number of studies,

including one conducted by scientists at Erasmus University Rotterdam that tested how writing down, clarifying, and planning long-term goals would affect the academic performance of college students.[1]

This was mediated through an online writing exercise that asked the students, who ranged from top-of-class to bottom-percentile performers, to explain why they were going to school, and how they were going to make the most of the opportunity.

The students answered questions like . . .

- "What would you like to learn more about, in the next six months? Two years? Five years?"
- "What habits would you like to improve?"
- "Where do you want to be in six months? Two years? Five years? Why? What are you trying to accomplish?"

Then, they were instructed to prioritize their goals, break them into subgoals, and create a list of potential barriers and ways to deal with them should they arise.

One year later, the researchers reviewed the progress of the participants, and the results were striking. Every single group of participants earned more college credits and were more likely to stay in school after their first year, and most surprising were the results seen with ethnic minority students, who earned 44 percent more college credits and were 54 percent more likely to remain enrolled.

Keep in mind that this exercise wasn't difficult, either. It didn't take much time, effort, or thought, yet it produced the kind of results that can be the difference between leaving school and landing a high-paying job versus languishing around the poverty line.

(In case you were wondering, this exercise was the Self

Authoring Program, which you can learn about in the free bonus materials you can download at www.workoutmotivationbook. com/bonus.)

A good first step for crystallizing our wishes is asking of them, "How will I know when I have succeeded?"

For example, "I want to lose weight" might turn into "I want to fit into my size-five jeans," "I want to be healthier" might turn into "I want to have normal blood pressure and cholesterol levels," and for a woman, "I want to get fit" might turn into "I want to gain ten pounds of muscle and reduce my body fat to 20 percent."

From here, the common recommendations to strength-en your commitment and follow-through mirror the general approach of the writing exercise outlined above: write down your goals, make a plan, make sure the first couple of milestones are easy, anticipate barriers, track your progress, either in terms of how far you've come or how much you have left (focus on whichever is smaller), and reward yourself as you make headway.

These are all valid and valuable tactics, but before you do any of that, you first need to reflect on another question:

"What kind of pain do I want?"

Stating a desire is easy, and especially when it's something everybody wants, like a better body, more time and freedom, or more income or savings. The hard part is taking the stars out of our eyes and considering how much pain we're willing to endure to get these things. The pain of sacrifice, tedium, doubt, disappointment, and despair. The pain that can shatter self-con-fidence, stifle self-expression, and squash self-actualization.

This means that before committing ourselves to a reward, we have to first assess the cost and see if we're willing to pay it. If we're going to have any chance at success, we have to first face the terrain that lies ahead before setting out to traverse it.

Tom Brady will go down in football history as one of the greatest quarterbacks to ever play the game, but many years ago, he was just "Tommy," a ninth-grader who wasn't good enough to even start on a team that finished 0–8 and didn't score a single touchdown.

Most people in the young Brady's life thought baseball was his best sport, and so didn't understand his decision to play football instead. He had an arm, but he wasn't fast, he wasn't agile, and he spent his first season warming the bench. Where could this possibly go?

Brady paid them no mind. "One day, I'm going to be a household name," he wrote in a school paper. His family had a good laugh. As much as they loved and supported Tommy, they never could have even dreamed that "The Little Brady," as many people knew him, would one day join the ranks of legends like Joe Montana and Johnny Unitas.

How did he do it? It's rather simple, really. He gave up everything to become great at football.

As Brady said in his 2018 six-part Facebook Watch documentary *Tom vs. Time*, "What are you willing to do, and what are you willing to give up to be the best you can be? You only have so much energy, and the clock ticks on all of us."

"If you're going to compete against me," he added, "you better be willing to give up your life, because I'm giving up mine."

That's the spirit that inspired Tommy to do things teenagers didn't normally do, like devise his own grueling jump-rope program to improve his footwork, do evening workouts after school and homework instead of playing video games, and obsessively practice a tedious hopscotch-like exercise that his teammates hated and cursed called the "five-dot drill."

That's the spirit that inhabits all extraordinary performers. That's what it all comes down to.

For example, Thomas Edison's lifelong, defining goal was to discover the secrets of nature and exploit them for the happiness of humankind. Every lesser goal—every invention of his—was merely an offshoot of that one, perennial, unquenchable ambition that embraced the entire world and human race.

Like Edison, Marie Curie's goals also forged her identity. She was once a young governess with a burning passion to leave Poland and study science in Paris, as women weren't permitted an advanced education in her home country. This was beyond the means of her family, however, so she arranged a deal with her sister, Bronya, whereby Marie would tutor children to help pay for Bronya's education, and once Bronya had graduated, the favor would be repaid.

For nearly three years, Marie spent her days working to cover her sister's costs and spent her nights alone, at her desk, reading outdated volumes on sociology, physics, and mathematics without guidance or advice—studies that she later said were "encompassed with difficulty." But her perseverance paid off, and at twenty-four years old, after her sister had graduated from the Sorbonne and married, Marie was able to pursue her dream.

Marie's university studies were incredibly challenging due to a deficient secondary education. She overcame her academic shortcomings, however, in glorious fashion by ultimately winning a Nobel Prize—the first woman to do so—for her doctoral thesis on radioactivity, which was an immensely difficult subject only recently discovered. Eight years later, she won a second Nobel Prize, the first person to do so, this time for her research into radium and polonium.

Aristotle honored this way of life in his elegant formula for success and happiness. "First," he wrote, "have a definite, clear practical ideal; a goal, an objective. Second, have the necessary means to achieve your ends; wisdom, money, materials, and methods. Third, adjust all your means to that end."

We're often told that the failure to achieve goals is due to a lack of motivation, passion, or some other elusive feeling. We're often told that we just need to think bigger or deeper, to hitch our wagons to a star and meditate on what success looks like and what we really want to achieve.

Failure is rarely solved along these lines. Instead, you have to embody your answer to the question Brady has been answering every day for the last twenty-five years: what are you willing to give up?

When you view objectives in this light, you quickly learn that effective goal setting is more a matter of effective goal *selection* than anything else. In other words, you must first decide which goals are worth the pain and which aren't, and then focus all of your attention and efforts on the things in the first bucket, and abandon the rest.

As Ray Dalio says in *Principles*, "I learned that if you work hard and creatively, you can have just about anything you want, but not everything you want. Maturity is the ability to reject good alternatives in order to pursue even better ones."

If you don't do this—if you try to push yourself in too many directions toward too many goals—you'll experience what psychologists refer to as "goal competition."

Your goals will compete with each other for your time and attention, and the thinner you try to slice these resources, the more frayed and frazzled they (and you) will become. This is why less is often more with goal setting, and why you must be brutally honest with yourself about what you're truly willing to pay to have the things you say you want.

Imagine your life is represented by a stove that's fueled by your time and effort, and that your goals are meals you want to cook on the stove.

You only have so many burners to work with, and you can only burn so much fuel for so long before, well, burning out, so you have a choice to make: do you bring a smaller number of meals to completion before starting others, or do you try to cook a dozen meals simultaneously by rotating them on and off the range in a frenzied act of culinary juggling?

You don't have to know much about cooking to know that while the latter approach might eventually turn out food, you're probably not going to want to eat most of it.

So it goes in life. You only have so much bandwidth. While it's possible to work toward a smorgasbord of long-term goals every day on several fronts—health, hobbies, work, family, and friends, for example—it requires a singular capacity for sustained effort and resilience in the face of hardship, and an outsized appetite for disorder and chaos. And even then, it takes its toll.

A smarter approach to goal setting and striving, then, relies on specification, prioritization, and elimination—on clarifying exactly what we want, identifying the prices we're willing to pay, choosing the most important objectives of the lot, and focusing intently on them.

There are many methods out there for this, but one I particularly like is Warren Buffett's "2 List Strategy," which was introduced to me by my friend James Clear.

As the most successful investor of the twentieth century and one of the world's richest men, Buffett needs no introduction. It goes without saying that we can all learn something from him on how to better set and achieve goals.

Buffett's strategy is particularly brilliant, because it can be applied to overarching life goals, domain-specific goals, and even weekly to-do lists. It goes as follows:

STEP 1

Write down your top twenty-five goals, projects, or tasks.

Take your time, and get everything down that you feel drawn toward in general or in specific areas of your life.

Remember, hundreds of scientific experiments involving dozens of types of tasks and thousands of participants have proven conclusively that the more specific and challenging the goals are, the better the resulting performance, so be as specific as you can here.

Don't set vague goals that can't be measured, like "to do my best" or "to work hard." Push yourself to envision specific, challenging goals, like, "to win the XYZ award" or "to create product X by January 1."

STEP 2

Circle the top five most important goals, projects, or tasks of the twenty-five.

To determine which you should ultimately choose, start by circling the ones that stand out as the most critical, rewarding, or interesting.

Then, starting with the first of those, think about and write down the three biggest obstacles you might face in trying to accomplish it.

Who or what might get in your way? What might make it strenuous? What might you be required to sacrifice?

Now write down a few sentences about how it will feel to accomplish this goal, project, or task. What positive changes might occur in your life? What might make it worth it?

Now compare the negative and positive aspects of the goal, project, or task, and take your temperature regarding it. If you feel confident and energized, then keep it on your list. If you feel discouraged, or undecided, however, consider reformulating the goal or dropping it altogether.

Repeat this process for each of the goals, projects, or tasks you first circled, replacing those you've decided against with "next best" options.

Last, review the circled items that remain after the vetting, and from those, circle (again) the five that stand out as the most critical, rewarding, or interesting.

STEP 3
Separate these goals into two lists.

The top five goals, projects, or tasks comprise List A, and the rest comprise List B.

The next part is crucial. Instead of doing what most people would do—start working on List A as the primary focus and chip away at List B when time permits—Buffett says you should start working on List A and avoid everything on List B as a potential distraction until List A is complete.

Buffett approaches his goals in this fashion because he knows that everything takes more time, energy, and attention than we realize going in, and especially things that we care about. He does it this way because it's far easier and more enjoyable to sprint toward five dones than twenty-something half-dones.

Furthermore, it reduces the chances of things going catastrophically wrong—of Murphy's law manifesting itself—by reducing the amount of time it takes to get to done. Remember: the longer it takes to bring something into being, the more ways it can falter and fail.

It turns out that overachievers from all walks and disciplines of life have been doing this for a very long time. It turns out that this is one of the great "secrets" of greatness.

Recommended Reading
The ONE Thing by Gary Keller and Jay Papasan

Do This Now

Do the Buffett "2 List" exercise by considering the following five key areas of your life and writing down your top twenty-five goals, projects, or tasks.

1. Health
2. Work
3. Love
4. Family
5. Friends

Next, zero in on the five among the twenty-five that stand out as the most critical, rewarding, or interesting, and highlight them. Why are these your top five? Explain in writing.

Next, write down the three biggest obstacles that might get in the way of each of these goals. What might make them hard? What might you be required to sacrifice?

Now write down a few sentences about how it will feel to accomplish each of these goals, projects, or tasks. What positive changes might occur? What might make it worth it?

Now compare the negative and positive aspects of the goals, projects, or tasks, and take your temperature regarding them.

Keep those you feel confident and energized about, and reformulate or replace those you feel discouraged or undecided about with worthy alternatives.

CHAPTER SIX

How to Not Suck at Achieving Your Goals

"Life is one long battle; we have to fight at every step; and Voltaire very rightly says that if we succeed, it is at the point of the sword, and that we die with the weapon in our hand."
—Arthur Schopenhauer

Y ou know what you want to do. You've sharpened your focus, set your goals, and checked them twice.

Now what? How do you best go from *wanting* to *doing* to *done*?

Forget *Think and Grow Rich* and *The Secret*. No matter how many times you say you're going to make a million dollars or attract the body you want, you're going to have to put on your gloves and get into the ring.

As Dan Pink says in his outstanding 2012 book *To Sell Is Human*, we should ignore Napoleon Hill and listen to Bob the

Builder instead. Yes, the overalls-clad, hard-hat-sporting cartoon character with an abiding fetish for fixing things.

Bob doesn't spend his time chanting affirmations or cultivating his dream board. He's all about business. Here's the thing. Here's the objective. How are we going to get this done?

Research conducted by scientists at the University of Illinois and University of Southern Mississippi shows that this interrogative style of self-talk can trump wishful thinking, because it elicits answers that help you translate misty ambitions into concrete systems—into specific actions that, if repeated enough, will produce the desired results.[1]

Even the loftiest of goals can be processed in this way. No matter the ambition, there is a knowable and doable system that will get you there. Chances are something just like it has already been done many times before by many different people. Chances are you can follow in their footsteps.

Systems don't have to be complicated, either. In fact, the simpler a system is and the more it's rooted in fundamentals, the more likely it is to actually work.

For example, if you want to lose a significant amount of weight, your system needs just one moving part: energy balance. If you want to take that a step further and transform your body composition, then you only have to add a couple of levers, namely macronutrient balance and resistance training. Still, a rather simple system.

If you want to read a book every month, then all your system needs to produce is ten pages of reading per day, which takes most people about fifteen minutes.

If you want to earn more money, then chances are your system needs to help you upgrade just one or two skills that will allow you to produce and sell more valuable work.

When you look at it this way, systems help you bear the

burden of goals. The moment you concoct a goal, you've chosen to leave the warmth and comfort of where you are and what you know and journey into the cold, dark unknown. And if you're going to survive the trek to the summit of the mountain you've fixed your gaze on, then you're going to need a system for making your way. Your system is going to be the fire stick that keeps you warm, the compass that keeps you oriented, and the cross that keeps you hopeful.

Systems, my friend, are how to not suck at achieving your goals, and one of the easiest ways to build better systems is to shift your perspective toward probabilistic thinking. To understand why, let's start by considering a simple puzzle presented in Daniel Kahneman's groundbreaking 2013 book *Thinking, Fast and Slow*:

> *Tom W is a graduate student at the main university in your state. Please rank the following nine fields of graduate specialization in order of the likelihood that Tom W is now a student in each of these fields. Use 1 for the most likely, 9 for the least likely.*
>
> *Business administration*
> *Computer science*
> *Engineering*
> *Humanities and education*
> *Law*
> *Medicine*
> *Library science*
> *Physical and life sciences*
> *Social science and social work*

This question is easy to solve, because the only information you need is the relative size of enrollment in each of the fields.

As far as you know, Tom W was picked at random from the students, like a single gumball from a bowl. To decide whether the gumball is more likely to be blue or yellow, you simply need to know how many gumballs of each color there are in the bowl. The proportion of one color to the others is called a *base rate*.

Similarly, the base rate of one graduate specialization or another is the proportion of students in it among all of the graduate students. Therefore, without additional information about Tom, you'd be correct to guess his likelihood of specialization conforms to the base rates, which state, for example, that he's more likely to be enrolled in humanities and education than computer or library science, because the former groups contain more students than the latter ones.

This simple intellectual exercise has profound implications for how we live our lives, because whether we realize it or not, every decision we make, both big and small, has different base rates associated with myriad different outcomes, both good and bad.

For example, the more a human being smokes cigarettes, the more his base rate of developing cardiovascular disease and cancer rises; the more time he spends on social media, the more his base rate of experiencing depression and anxiety rises; and the more overweight he is, the more his base rate of developing type 2 diabetes rises.

By the same token, the more time he spends in deliberate practice of a commercially viable skill, the more his base rate of achieving financial success rises; the more consecutive days he sticks to his diet and exercise program, the more his base rate of achieving his fitness goals rises; and the more often he goes to church and connects with his community, the more his base rate of experiencing more personal happiness rises.

Base rates are just the starting point for predictions, too, because when other factors enter the picture, probabilities change. In the case of Tom, if I were to give you insights into his character that made him clearly more suited to one or more fields of specializations than others, you would adjust your estimations accordingly.

In the same way, the ultimate impact of smoking, social media, and body fatness on your physical and mental health will depend in part on many genetic and lifestyle factors. Some people's deliberate practice is likely to be more fruitful than others', some people's bodies are likely to respond better or worse to dieting, and some people tend to derive more or less enjoyment from socializing.

This means, then, that the general quality of any aspect of our lives is mostly determined by the quality of the many decisions we've made that have affected and are affecting it—the quality of our systems (or lack thereof).

If we don't have the body we want, it's probably because we decided too many times to "cheat" on our diets and skip workouts. If we don't make enough money, it's probably because we decided too many times to do things other than working to cultivate and capitalize on marketable skills. If we don't have a good social life, it's probably because we decided too many times to avoid or undermine friendships.

This is a tough row to hoe for most people. They want to do whatever they want to do in the day-to-day without ever considering the bigger picture—what kind of character and life they're cobbling together. As Carl Jung once said, "Until you make the unconscious conscious, it will direct your life and you will call it fate."

And if these people do happen to reflect on what might ultimately result from their choices, they often grossly and unjustifiably distort base rates to fit the stories they want to believe. They convince themselves that both the good and bad decisions they make are far better than they really are, and that the rewards will far outweigh the penalties.

"Things will probably work out fine in the end," they say, when in fact, the exact opposite is true—probabilistically speaking, things will probably *not* turn out well, and if they do, it will be against long odds.

And so many people regularly engage in activities that are not only unlikely to produce meaningful value at any point in their lives, but are probably just going to make things worse by making them unhealthier, weaker, lazier, dumber, and generally less alive and less effective.

A good analogy for all of this is gambling. We enter the casino of life at a young age with an enormous but finite amount of resources to play with in the form of time, attention, and effort. This casino has many different games we can play and many different rewards we can win. Our goal is simple: to win as much as we can at as many of the games as we can. How do we do this?

By choosing our games wisely and then developing a system that allows us to make more winning than losing bets, or making sure our winning bets are much larger than our losing bets. And how do we do that?

By developing an ability to weigh the size of wagers against the potential payoffs and probabilities of winning (*expected value* in gambling parlance).

Let's say you're playing the game of building a healthier, stronger body, and you can wager a few hundred hours of time, attention, and effort on proper diet and exercise, and be more or less guaranteed to win. Is that a good bet? I'd say so.

Or let's say you're playing the game of money making, and you can wager a thousand hours of your time to develop a skill set that can command six figures in annual income with significant potential for future growth. Furthermore, because it suits your intelligence, personality, and talents, you figure you have at least a 50 percent chance of winning. Is that a good bet? You'd be silly to pass it up.

When viewed through this lens, many of the bets (decisions) people make every day have such a poor expected value that you can only wonder if they even understand what games they're playing, let alone the systems they're employing. Drug and alcohol abuse, countless hours of social media, internet browsing, and TV watching, sedentary living, intellectual stagnation, and egregious overeating and overspending come immediately to mind, but I'm sure you can think of many other examples.

So then, how do we go about building effective systems that make it easier to make the right bets in our lives?

Well, one of my favorite formulas for this has just three components:

1. What, When, Where, If, Then
2. Shut Up Until You've Put Up
3. Let's Get Accountable

Let's take a closer look at each.

What, When, Where, If, Then

What if I told you that filling out one simple little sentence could increase your chances of achieving a goal by 100 to 200 percent?

What if this sentence worked subconsciously to automatically reduce your need for motivation, willpower, or self-control?

And what if you could use this sentence for all types of goals, including exercise, diet, health, and everything else?

Thanks to the work of a number of psychologists over the

course of a decade, this sentence exists, and it has three parts: what, when, and where.

This sentence was the focus of a study conducted by researchers at the University of Bath, who randomly assigned 248 adults to one of three groups.[2]

1. People who were asked to read a few paragraphs from a random novel before working out.
2. People who were asked to read a pamphlet on the heart benefits of exercise, and were told that most young adults who stick to an exercise program reduce their risk of heart disease.
3. People who were also asked to read the pamphlet, but in addition, to use the following sentence to formulate an exact exercise plan: "During the next week, I will partake in at least twenty minutes of vigorous exercise on [DAY] at [TIME OF DAY] at/in [PLACE]."

Two weeks later, here's what the researchers found:

- Thirty-eight percent of participants in the first group exercised at least once per week.
- Thirty-five percent of participants in the second group exercised at least once per week.
- Ninety-one percent of participants in the third group exercised at least once per week.

No, that's not a typo. By simply writing when and where exercise was going to occur, follow-through skyrocketed.

Similar results have been seen in other exercise studies, as well as research analyzing a variety of positive behaviors ranging from breast self-examination to dietary adherence, condom usage, breast and cervical screenings, vitamin supplementation, alcohol intake, and more.[3]

As it happens, there are over one hundred published studies on this phenomenon, and the conclusion is crystal clear: if you explicitly state what you're going to do, when you're going to do it, and where you're going to do it, you're much more likely to actually do it.

For example:

- "Every Monday, Wednesday, and Friday, I'm going to wake up at 7 a.m., drink an espresso, and go to the gym" will be far more effective than "I'm going to start exercising."
- "Every evening after dinner, I'm going to sit on the balcony and read twenty-five pages before watching TV," and not "I'm going to read every day."
- "Every Friday after I deposit my paycheck, I'm going to go on my computer at home and transfer 10 percent of it into my savings account" will help you grow your savings a lot faster than "I'm going to save more than I did last year."

What–when–where statements are far more effective for regulating behavior than relying on inspiration or willpower to strike at the right moment, because they speak the brain's natural language, creating a trigger-and-response mechanism that doesn't require conscious monitoring or analysis.

If you want to get even more out of this process, you can include another type of statement that's scientifically proven to increase self-control: the if–then statement. Together, these two formulas can create powerful subconscious models for future behavior.

An if–then statement looks like this: If X happens, then I will do Y. This works for the same reason what–where–when statements work, and it allows you to plan for life's curveballs and contingencies and thereby reduce the need for self-control or willpower when things go sideways.

For example, let's say you have decided that every Monday, Wednesday, and Friday, you're going to wake up at 7 a.m., drink an espresso, and go to the gym. To generate complementary if–then statements, think about what might get in the way of your plan, and what you'll do in each scenario.

Here's a good start:

- If I don't get enough sleep, then I will still get up at 7 a.m. and do my workout.
- If I miss a workout for any reason, then I will do it after work.
- If I can't go to the gym after work, then I will do the workout on Saturday or Sunday at 9 a.m.

Every what–when–where statement can be strengthened in this way, and especially after you've gotten into action. Unforeseen obstacles and complications will require that you augment and adjust your systems, including the whats, whens, wheres, ifs, and thens.

Psychologists call this process of using mental exercises to stress test your desired outcomes "mental contrasting," and research conducted by scientists at the University of Hamburg, University of Freiburg, and New York University shows that it can increase your motivation to overcome obstacles and achieve your goals.[4]

Interestingly, it can also decrease your motivation, depending on how you respond to the process.

As the developer of this technique, Gabriele Oettingen, explained in her 2014 book *Rethinking Positive Thinking*, if you catalog all the potential barriers, snags, and stumbling blocks you can think of and still believe you can achieve your goal, you'll probably feel a surge of motivation. On the other hand, you might realize your goal is unrealistic ("Go from zero to playing Liszt's 'Campanella' in a few months") or simply not worth pursuing given the level of difficulty that you foresee.

Either way, the outcome is positive. You steam forward with even more clarity and confidence, or you go back to the drawing board and rework your vision into something more plausible.

Shut Up Until You've Put Up

In 1926, an anonymous millionaire known only as "RHJ" published a short book titled *It Works*.

The mysterious RHJ attributed all he had accomplished in his life—from amassing wealth, to overcoming great hardships, to winning loyal friends—to the three principles taught in his book.

The first step is very simple: Don't talk about your goals until you can show objective results.

The reason for this is twofold, he explains. First, it prevents the fear of what others might think if you fail, and second, it prevents you from feeling satisfied with yourself by merely talking about what you're "going to do" as opposed to actually doing it.

It turns out this is indeed a simple but powerful way to increase stick-to-itiveness.

Research conducted by scientists at New York University has shown that people who announce their intentions to others and receive acknowledgment are less likely to actually work to achieve those goals, and ironically, also tend to be strangely optimistic about their (lack of) progress.[5] Furthermore, people who don't announce their goals tend to work harder toward them, and to more realistically assess their progress.

For instance, in one study conducted by the same research team, first-year law students were asked to write down how much they wanted to succeed and what they were doing to achieve their goals.[5] Then, half of the participants were asked to share their goals with the group, while the other half was asked to share their opinions on some pictures (the control group).

Researchers found that the group that publicly shared their goals felt they were somehow closer to realizing them than the group that didn't.

The reason for this is telling people what you plan on doing can create a premature sense of accomplishment. Being admired for talking about something can feel just as good as being admired for doing it.

That said, while keeping everything we're up to completely under wraps does have its advantages, it's not very practical. Eventually, details are going to slip out to one person or another. And that's okay, because it turns out that complete radio silence isn't necessary.

In fact, discussing your goals with others in the right way can actually increase your chances of staying the course and succeeding.

When you're going to tell someone about what you're up to, do it in such a way that emphasizes your commitment to the goals, not what you're aiming for. In other words, indicate you're working on something with no implication of having arrived or achieved anything.

For example:

- "I'm working on losing twenty pounds" and not "I've joined a gym and go every morning!"
- "I'm trying to make my business profitable by the end of the year" and not "I've already made so-and-so much

sales this year!"
- "I'm learning another language" and not "I've already put a hundred hours into French!"

You know you've got it right when you don't get praise or approval, but instead a lukewarm "That's nice."

If you do this, you can learn to let go of the need for external approval, and in turn, the need for external motivation and positive reinforcement. If you can do this, you can become the type of person who makes plans, does the work, and lets their outcomes do the talking.

You can pay this forward too. Do the people in your life a favor, and don't fawn over their stated goals and intentions. When they share something they intend on doing, encourage them to do it. Praise is reserved for dones, not going-to-dos.

Let's Get Accountable

There's another way to talk about your goals that can markedly increase your chances of success, and it has to do with accountability.

In 2015, Dr. Gail Matthews of Dominican University presented findings of a study she had conducted to see how formulating, stating, and being accountable to goals ultimately affects one's success or failure.[6]

The study was conducted over a one-month period, and included 149 participants split into five groups:

1. People who simply thought about goals.
2. People who wrote down their goals.
3. People who wrote down their goals and formulated action   steps to reach them.

4. People who wrote down their goals, formulated action steps, and sent these steps to a friend.
5. People who wrote down their goals, formulated action steps, sent them to a friend, and created weekly reports on their progress, which they also sent to the friend.

The group of people who simply wrote down their goals was 44 percent more successful in accomplishing them than those in the first group—the people who just thought about their goals. Impressive, no doubt.

Until you hear the results of the fifth group, whose members wrote down goals, formulated action steps, sent them to a friend, and reported weekly on their progress. These people were 77 *percent* more successful in accomplishing their goals than the first group.

The findings of the study were clear: writing down specific goals, working out specific steps to achieve them, and creating accountability appear to be very conducive to success.

An easy way to put this research into practice is to recruit someone you love and trust to hold you accountable to your goals. Then, do the following:

1. Share your plans with them.
2. Commit to getting something specific and tangible done in the next week.
3. At the end of the week, reconnect and have them ask you if you did what you said you were going to do. If you did, you get a high-five. If you didn't, you get punched in the face.
4. Repeat steps 2 and 3.

Okay, so maybe you don't need to get punched for not keeping your word, but there should be unwanted consequences for not doing what you said you were going to do. Studies show that appealing to fear is a very effective way to influence attitude, intentions, and behaviors, so why not use that to your advantage?[7]

You can choose the form of punishment, but it has to be something that carries enough weight to make you think twice when temptation to stray strikes. The easiest way to achieve this is through money, because no matter how much you might have, there's always an amount that stings when lost.

A particularly popular financial punishment is leaving a meaningful amount of cash with your accountability partner with instructions to donate it to a cause or organization you despise should you fail to follow through with your weekly actions. (Remember www.stickk.com from the chapter on sacrifice?)

You now know more than most people ever will about formulating, prioritizing, and accomplishing goals, and are well equipped with effective strategies and tools for making your desires a reality.

Before we end our discussion on the matter, however, I want to leave you with a counterintuitive but powerful lesson I've learned:

The content of your goals—what you're striving for—isn't as important as many people think.

Most people know that it requires passion to accomplish anything extraordinary, but struggle to discover what makes them feel passionate. If only they could stumble on the right goals, they think, they would finally come alive and have what it takes to succeed.

This is backward. You can't search out passion; you can only create it.

People who are good at this can wonder at and get excited about many different things, large and small, and people who aren't can't be enthused under any circumstances.

This explains why some people have to roll themselves out of bed every day like a log off a truck to run multimillion-dollar enterprises, while others wake up every morning absolutely thrilled to run their pig farms or make pottery from cow poop. (Yup, that's a thing.)

Something tells me that fate isn't involved here—that the latter folk weren't dreaming of such activities when they were children. Instead, they learned to love their work. How?

Leonardo da Vinci was probably the ultimate embodiment of this principle. He was just as excited to create what would become the most famous painting in history—the Mona Lisa— as he was to dissect rotting corpses by candlelight to discover which facial muscles and nerves produced a smile.

The big "secret," I believe, is rather simple, and expressed by Mihaly Csikszentmihalyi in his landmark 2008 book *Flow*:

> *The peak of the mountain is important only because it justifies climbing, which is the real goal of the enterprise.*

In other words, a goal is only important insofar as it inspires energetic commitment and enables us to find meaning in the struggle along the way, which lasts an eternity compared to the fleeting moments in which we design our aims.

The real way to escape the rat race of chasing the fickle and finicky goddess of passion is to become the type of person who's less concerned with *what* they're striving for than with the *experience* of striving—the type of person who derives enjoyment from working to manifest any and all of their visions for the future, whether they're images of the ideal flowerbed or conceptions of revolutionary reform.

That isn't to say that we won't be naturally drawn toward certain goals and activities over others, or that we should ignore these affinities, but, rather, if our imaginations are robust enough, we should never want for attractive endeavors that stimulate our curiosities and feed our ambitions.

Recommended Reading
The Motivation Myth by Jeff Haden

Do This Now

Review the five goals, projects, or tasks you settled on at the end of the last chapter, and formulate and write down next actions (remember that from Chapter 3?) for each one, including what–when–where statements for each.

Next, write down at least one potential obstacle that might get in the way of each of these next actions, followed by if–then statements for dealing with each of the obstacles.

Next, it's time to set up an accountability partner for the five goals, projects, or tasks you wrote down in the last chapter.

To do that, think of someone you love and trust, and who will be supportive and not judgmental.

Ask if they will be your accountability partner, explaining how it works. Chances are they would love to. Then . . .

1. At the beginning of each week (which can start on a day of your choosing), specify the next actions that

you will complete within the next seven days.

2. At the end of each week, check in with your accountability partner and share if you did what you said you were going to.

3. If you didn't, you face a negative consequence. What could it be? Remember that financial penalties are an easy solution, and www.stickk.com is an easy tool for setting this up.

4. Repeat this process every week until you've accomplished your goals, projects, or tasks.

Have fun!

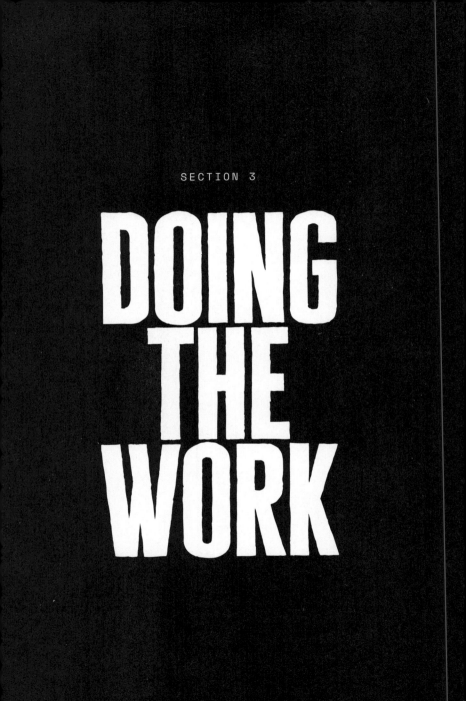

SECTION 3

DOING THE WORK

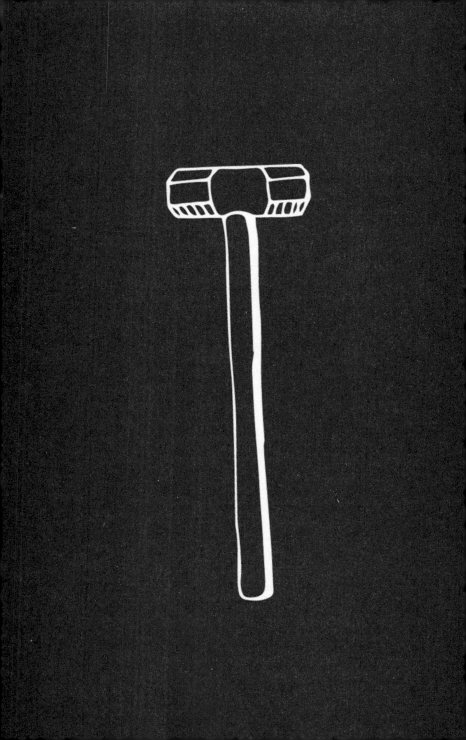

CHAPTER SEVEN

You Can Fight Resistance Now or Hate Yourself Later

"In this age, which believes that there is a shortcut to everything, the greatest lesson to be learned is that the most difficult way is, in the long run, the easiest."
—Henry Miller

"I'm really going to stick to my exercise and diet programs and completely change my body!" people say every day. "Oh man, I need to tweet about this before I forget."

Twitter is loaded, 280 characters are carefully crafted, and the proclamation is made.

"I probably should write a quick blog post about it," someone else muses.

A few hours later, a few hundred words are posted, and a few minutes are spent basking in the afterglow.

"I can't wait! I'm going to get so ripped. Wow. I should probably start looking at how I'm going to revamp my wardrobe—"

"ENOUGH!" a disembodied voice booms.

They snap to attention. "What?"

The reply is only three words.

"Do. The. Work."

"What?"

"DO THE WORK."

People share their health and fitness goals with me all the time. They have pretty spreadsheets, fancy workout plans, and fanciful visions of turning heads at the beach and posing in underwear ads.

My reply is always the same.

"That sounds good. It looks like it's time to do the work."

This is usually followed by an awkward silence.

"Well . . . yeah . . . I've been reading a bit more to make sure I haven't missed anything, and I've picked up some really good tips. I also am meeting with a couple trainers to see if I want to get some professional help, and I'm tweaking my one-year plan, which is looking really good. Here, let me show you—"

"No, I think you misunderstood me. It sounds like it's time to do the real work. The hard work. The work you don't want to do."

Another awkward silence.

They don't get it. Or they don't want to get it.

They aren't doing the work, and they won't succeed regardless of how busy they keep themselves with not doing it.

What's going on? It's simple. They're getting whipped in the war against Resistance.

Resistance is insidious and impersonal. It can't be seen, but it's swirling in you right now, and it can be felt. It will tell you anything to keep you from doing the work. It will lie, argue, bluster, seduce, and bully you to get its way. It will say anything to strike a deal, and then stab you in the back. It doesn't care who you are or what you want to do. It has no conscience.

What kinds of things does Resistance hate most? Any creative artistic action. Any type of entrepreneurial venture. Any new diet or fitness regimen. Any method of spiritual advancement. Any type of education. Anything courageous. In short, Resistance hates anything that requires you to forgo immediate gratification in search of long-term growth or fulfillment.

In his wildly popular 2011 book *The War of Art*, Steven Pressfield fingered Resistance as personal enemy number one, but he wasn't the first to do so. In 1904, Freud wrote that "psychoanalytic treatment may in general be conceived of as such a reeducation in overcoming internal resistances."

One of the many insights Pressfield shares on Resistance is its Achilles' heel: it will only fight that which is truly important in your life. It wants to kill your deepest purposes and desires, your true calling and gifts. Yes, kill them. By the same token, however, it also shows you what work you must do—your very personal path to profound fulfillment and success.

Resistance dares you to meet it in pitched battle. When you do anything but the work, it sneers. It's playing you like a marionette. When you do the work, though, it shrieks in horror. "Anything but the work!" it cries. It counterattacks by invading your mind and shouting catcalls. Television! Video games! Social media! ANYTHING BUT THE WORK!

Make no mistake. The fight against Resistance is a war to the death. It will tell you you're too weak to win. Too stupid. Too lazy. But you're not. Ironically, it depends on your obedience for its strength. It can only overpower you and win if you let it.

Defiantly do the work instead, though, and Resistance withers. Every bit done strikes at it. Do enough work, and eventually its armor crumbles, its power fades, and all that's left is a whispering ghost. Do even more work, and it even stops whispering.

If you're trying to create a healthy, strong, vital body, a business, a career, a relationship, or anything else positive in your life, you're a warrior, and your primary enemy is Resistance.

Remember this when you're going for the snooze button, when you're procrastinating in the parking lot, and when you're struggling through a tough workout. Remember it when getting into the gym is the last thing you want to do, when you're groping for an excuse to skip, because that's often a sign it's exactly what you should do.

Remember too that Future You is depending on Present You. Every day, you're faced with one of two decisions: sell yourself a little further down the river, or do the work now and realize your potential. Put if off today, and you'll be more likely to procrastinate tomorrow. Get into action now, and tomorrow will be easier.

So don't give in to the siren song of "fair-weather fitness." Put in the work, even when it's hard, and you'll be rewarded with something far better than fleeting comfort: *satisfaction*.

The satisfaction of knowing that you're closing the day a little closer to your aims, that you're living up to your standards, that you have what it takes to do what it takes.

So while you may not enjoy every workout, remember that you're always going to enjoy having worked out.

Every day you show up to grunt, groan, and grind is another day on the front lines in the battle against Resistance. With every rep, set, and session, you gain a little more ground and earn a few more of your stripes.

Recommended Reading
The War of Art by Steven Pressfield

Do This Now

The first step to defeating Resistance is becoming aware of it, and that's what this exercise is going to do: increase your awareness of the Resistance you face in your life.

For the next seven days, every time you run into Resistance in any task or activity, write down what you were doing that triggered it, how it manifested and made you feel, and what you did as a result (good or bad).

After this week of journaling, review your entries to see if anything insightful jumps out at you.

Are there any discernible patterns among the things that sparked the Resistance, like people, places, or situations? If so, could you take any actions to avoid those things going forward?

Also, if you'd like to tap into some "crowd wisdom" and speak with positive, supportive, like-minded people who are striving to become the best they can be, join my Facebook group, which you can find here:

www.facebook.com/groups/muscleforlife

This group is chock-full of people who can answer your questions, push you forward, cheer your victories, and soothe your setbacks, and for whom you can do the same in return.

All you have to do is visit the link above, then tap the "+ Join" button. One of my team members will approve your application, and you'll be ready to go.

CHAPTER EIGHT

Can You Carry a Message to Garcia?

"Today is victory over yourself of yesterday; tomorrow is your victory over lesser men."
—Miyamoto Musashi

n February 22, 1899, a businessman named Elbert Hubbard sat down after a long, trying day at work, and in an hour, scribbled an essay to vent his frustrations.

The essay relates the quest of a lieutenant named Rowan, whom his son believed was the real hero of the Spanish–American war. If Rowan hadn't delivered a message to a general named Garcia, the son claimed, Teddy Roosevelt may never have charged his Rough Riders up the San Juan Hill and achieved fame and victory, and Cuba may never have achieved independence from Spain.

Hubbard's article recounted Lieutenant Rowan's story and passionately argued that it's people like him who keep the motor of the world running.

At the time, Hubbard published a small magazine called *The Philistine*, and he thought so little of his Rowan commentary that he ran it without a heading. Soon after the edition went out, orders for more copies began to come in. And then more, larger orders began to come in. And then the American News Corporation requested one thousand copies.

Hubbard was flabbergasted at the unprecedented demand for his publication, and asked his team which article had stirred the cosmic dust.

"It's the stuff about Garcia," one of his employees told him.

The very next day, a telegram arrived at Hubbard's desk from an officer at the New York Central Railroad, asking for the price of one hundred thousand pamphlets of "the Rowan article" and how quickly they could be shipped.

This turned into multiple editions of over five hundred thousand copies each, and by 1913, millions of copies of what came to be known as *A Message to Garcia* had been printed, and it had appeared in hundreds of magazines and newspapers and been translated into scores of other languages; it continues to sell to this very day.

I want to share this 1,474-word article with you, because I believe all of us should aspire to be the type of person who can carry a message to Garcia.

A Message to Garcia
By Elbert Hubbard

In all this Cuban business there is one man stands out on the horizon of my memory like Mars at perihelion.

When war broke out between Spain and the United States,

it was very necessary to communicate quickly with the leader of the Insurgents. Garcia was somewhere in the mountain fastnesses of Cuba—no one knew where. No mail or telegraph could reach him. The President must secure his co-operation, and quickly.

What to do!

Someone said to the President, "There's a fellow by the name of Rowan will find Garcia for you, if anybody can."

Rowan was sent for and given a letter to be delivered to Garcia. How "the fellow by name of Rowan" took the letter, sealed it up in an oilskin pouch, strapped it over his heart, in four days landed by night off the coast of Cuba from an open boat, disappeared into the jungle, and in three weeks came out on the other side of the island, having traversed a hostile country on foot, and having delivered his letter to Garcia, are things I have no special desire now to tell in detail. The point I wish to make is this: McKinley gave Rowan a letter to be delivered to Garcia; Rowan took the letter and did not ask, "Where is he at?"

By the Eternal! There is a man whose form should be cast in deathless bronze and the statue placed in every college in the land. It is not book-learning young men need, nor instruction about this or that, but a stiffening of the vertebrae which will cause them to be loyal to a trust, to act promptly, concentrate their energies; do the thing—"Carry a message to Garcia!"

General Garcia is dead now, but there are other Garcias. No man, who has endeavored to carry out an enterprise where many hands were needed, but has been well-nigh appalled at times by the imbecility of the average man—the inability or unwilling-ness to concentrate on a thing and do it.

Slipshod assistance, foolish inattention, dowdy indifference, and half-hearted work seem the rule; and no man succeeds, unless by hook or crook, or threat, he forces or bribes other men to assist him; or mayhap, God in His goodness performs a miracle, and sends him an Angel of Light for an assistant.

You, reader, put this matter to a test: You are sitting now in your office—six clerks are within your call. Summon anyone and make this request: "Please look in the encyclopedia and make a brief memorandum for me concerning the life of Correggio."

Will the clerk quietly say, "Yes, sir," and go do the task?

On your life, he will not. He will look at you out of a fishy eye, and ask one or more of the following questions:

Who was he?

Which encyclopedia?

Where is the encyclopedia?

Was I hired for that?

Don't you mean Bismarck?

What's the matter with Charlie doing it?

Is he dead?

Is there any hurry?

Shan't I bring you the book and let you look it up yourself?

What do you want to know for?

And I will lay you ten to one that after you have answered the questions, and explained how to find the information, and why you want it, the clerk will go off and get one of the two other clerks to help him find Garcia, and then come back and tell you there is no such man. Of course I may lose my bet, but according to the Law of Average, I will not.

Now if you are wise you will not bother to explain to your "assistant" that Correggio is indexed under the C's, not in the K's; but you will smile sweetly and say: "Never mind," and go look it up yourself. And this incapacity for independent action, this moral stupidity, this infirmity of the will, this unwilling-ness to cheerfully catch hold and lift, are the things that put pure socialism so far into the future. If men will not act for themselves, what will they do when the benefit of their effort is for all?

A first mate with knotted club seems necessary; and the dread of getting "the bounce" Saturday night holds many a worker in his place.

Advertise for a stenographer, and nine times out of ten who apply can neither spell nor punctuate—and do not think it necessary to.

Can such a one write a letter to Garcia?

"You see that bookkeeper," said the foreman to me in a large factory.

"Yes, what about him?"

"Well, he's a fine accountant, but if I'd send him to town on an errand, he might accomplish the errand all right, and, on the other hand, might stop at four saloons on the way, and when he got to Main Street, would forget what he had been sent for."

Can such a man be entrusted to carry a message to Garcia?

We have recently been hearing much maudlin sympathy expressed for the "downtrodden denizen of the sweat shop" and the "homeless wanderer searching for honest employment," and with it all often go many hard words for the men in power.

Nothing is said about the employer who grows old before his time in a vain attempt to get frowsy ne'er-do-wells to do intelligent work; and his long patient striving with "help" that does nothing but loaf when his back is turned. In every store and factory there is a constant weeding-out process going on. The employer is constantly sending away "help" that have shown their incapacity to further the interests of the business, and others are being taken on. No matter how good times are, this sorting continues, only if times are hard and work is scarce, this sorting is done finer—but out and forever out, the incompetent and unworthy go. It is the survival of the fittest. Self-interest prompts every employer to keep the best—those who can carry a message to Garcia.

I know one man of really brilliant parts who has not the ability to manage a business of his own, and yet who is absolutely worthless to anyone else, because he carries with him constantly the insane suspicion that his employer is oppressing, or intending to oppress, him. He can not give orders, and he will not receive them. Should a message be given him to take to Garcia, his answer would probably be, "Take it yourself."

Tonight this man walks the streets looking for work, the wind whistling through his threadbare coat. No one who knows him dare employ him, for he is a regular firebrand of discontent. He is impervious to reason, and the only thing that can impress him is the toe of a thick-soled No. 9 boot.

Of course I know that one so morally deformed is no less to be pitied than a physical cripple; but in your pitying, let us drop a tear, too, for the men who are striving to carry on a great enterprise, whose working hours are not limited by the whistle, and whose hair is fast turning white through the struggle to hold the line in dowdy indifference, slipshod imbecility, and the heartless ingratitude which, but for their enterprise, would be both hungry and homeless.

Have I put the matter too strongly? Possibly I have; but when all the world has gone a-slumming I wish to speak a word of sympathy for the man who succeeds—the man who, against great odds, has directed the efforts of others, and, having succeeded, finds there's nothing in it: nothing but bare board and clothes. I have carried a dinner-pail and worked for a day's wages, and I have also been an employer of labor, and I know there is something to be said on both sides. There is no excellence, per se, in poverty; rags are no recommendation; and all employers are not rapacious and high-handed, any more than all poor men are virtuous.

My heart goes out to the man who does his work when the "boss" is away, as well as when he is home. And the man who, when given a letter for Garcia, quietly takes the missive, without asking any idiotic questions, and with no lurking intention of chucking it into the nearest sewer, or of doing aught else but deliver it, never gets "laid off," nor has to go on strike for higher wages. Civilization is one long anxious search for just such individuals. Anything such a man asks will be granted; his kind is so rare that no employer can afford to let him go. He is wanted in every city, town, and village—in every office, shop, store and factory. The world cries out for such; he is needed, and needed badly—the man who can carry a message to Garcia.

Something tells me this commentary wouldn't get many "claps" on Medium or retweets on Twitter.

You might find it objectionable yourself, instinctively pushing back against its stark language and harsh tone. If that feels like you, I challenge you to not dismiss it just yet.

First, consider this:

If you can carry a message to Garcia like Lieutenant Rowan did, you'll never want for work, praise, or achievement. If you can just do the thing, whatever it is and whatever may come, employers will beg for you, peers will marvel at you, and posterity will remember you as someone cut from a different cloth.

If you can carry a message to Garcia, you'll be the type of person who's reliable, responsible, and resolute. The type of person who doesn't just make noise, but who can do the hard thinking and work required to, as Buckminster Fuller famously said, "build a new model that makes the existing model obsolete." The type of person who has earned the right to be respected.

Hubbard's essay also alludes to the fact that, like its delivery, the most effective people are very often rough around the edges. A little savage, even. Not savage in the sense of evil or bullying, but in the sense of intense and aggressive.

The influential psychologist William James once said that, "We are all ready to be savage in some cause. The difference between a good man and a bad one is the choice of the cause."

Working out allows us to tap into this animalistic side. You have to be a little savage to push, pull, and squat crushing amounts of weight. You have to be a little fierce to go in for a WOD that might leave your lunch on the floor. You have to be a little relentless to run until your lungs and legs are ablaze.

It takes more than "inspiration," "motivation," and "positivity" to push our bodies to their limits. It takes ferocity. And that's also what it takes to carry a message to Garcia.

This is why I often think about my relationship with savagery. I think about it when I'm waking up at 5:30 a.m. to train and then start my ten-plus-hour workday. I think about it when I'm doing bicycle sprints later that night, gasping for air. I think about it when I'm showering in ice cold water, when I'm crunched on a deadline, running on fumes, and even when I'm taking a breather, recovering for the next blitz.

I think about savagery because in many competitions, you don't have to be the best to win. You just have to be harder to destroy.

Do you know why bulldogs were such formidable opponents in nineteenth-century dog fighting? It's not because they were the strongest or most agile or hostile of breeds, but because the extra fat and skin around their necks made it harder to rip their throats out. Other dogs had to work overtime to kill them. That's savage. And illustrative.

When you're indefatigable, when you can absorb a tremendous number of blows to get into the pole position, and when you can learn to embrace and even crave that process, you're a savage, and while you may not win every tilt, you're going to bat a lot better than average.

Recommended Reading
Do the Work by Steven Pressfield

Do This Now

Revisit the role model(s) you wrote in Chapter 4, and reflect on (or find out if you don't know) what they had to do and overcome to carry their messages to Garcia.

What feats did they pull off against long odds? Where did they refuse to give up? Who did they refuse to let stop them? Explain in writing, and then describe how you can apply these lessons to your life.

Specifically, write down one small-sized way you can begin to model their behavior in your own in the next week, and then one medium-sized way you can model their behavior in the next month.

For example, let's talk about one of my favorite characters in history, Alexander the Great.

Here's a guy who took about fifty thousand troops and went on a truly epic journey: he marched them thousands of miles to the ends of the known world and led them to victory in scores of sieges, battles, and skirmishes, including many where they were outnumbered several times over, and ultimately toppled the Persian empire and created what is still one of the largest kingdoms ever. Simply because he could.

In one of those battles, Alexander was attacking a city that belonged to one of the fiercest tribes in the Punjab region of India, the Malli.

The Indians had already lost several battles with the Macedonians and were making their last stand in the strongest of their fortresses. Alexander's soldiers tried to find a way into the citadel but couldn't breach the walls, so he grabbed a ladder and scaled the wall himself, followed by three of his men, and then fought his way through the defenders and jumped into the city and continued fighting alongside his bodyguard and attendant.

Meanwhile, his army was going berserk, frantically trying to gain entry to the stronghold before they lost their king. Inside, Alexander was struck by an arrow in the chest, but he continued to defend himself until collapsing from blood loss, with only two men and their shields to protect him from the rocks and arrows raining down.

Finally, the Macedonians shouldering the gates shattered the wooden bar holding them shut, and burst through just in time to save Alexander's life. They brought a litter to transfer him to a nearby ship for treatment, but in a final display of grit and glory, the king ordered a horse instead, clambered onto it, and rode through his ranks to reassure them that he wasn't going to die.

Here's how professor and historian Philip Freeman described the scene in his entertaining 2011 book *Alexander the Great*:

> Once he had regained some of his strength, his officers began
> to chide him that his performance on the wall was a brave but
> foolish act for a king. It was not the job of a commander, they
> said, to risk his life in such a way when there were plenty of
> men in the army who could do the same thing. Alexander did

not know how to tell his friends that for him such actions were an essential part of being a king. Faced with such criticism, he walked out of his tent into the camp. A grizzled veteran from Boeotia in central Greece who had heard about the rebukes of Alexander's companions approached him. The man looked the king straight in the eye and said just a few words in his rural dialect—'Alexander, brave deeds are what true men do.' The king embraced the old soldier and considered him a friend for the rest of his life.

My takeaway is the final beat in this story. Why did Alexander insist on taking such risks? Because that's what true men did, and that's the type of person he wanted to be.

After reading this, I wondered what type of person *I* wanted to be? What are *my* core values? I reflected on this question, and came up with the following list:

- Achievement
- Commitment
- Consistency
- Courage
- Creativity
- Education
- Enthusiasm
- Honesty
- Responsibility

I want to be able to confidently say that, through my actions, I'm the type of person who values those things the most.

As a result of this, while I've definitely had my share of ups and downs, I've also been able to keep my life on a generally upward trajectory by making a lot more good decisions than bad, and I expect things to continue improving as long as I stay true to who I want to be.

If I were to abandon those principles, though, and start living for the types of things that most people fantasize about—money, fame, physical pleasure, and the like—then I would become the type of person I really have no respect for, which would most certainly lead to my downfall. I keep this in mind when tempted to go astray, and it has helped me avoid people, situations, and decisions that would have almost certainly created problems not worth having.

So, back to the exercise: the next step is coming up with a small way I can start modeling Alexander's behavior—living with the courage of my convictions—in the next week.

Easy: start waking up earlier so I can get in some extra reading (*Education*) before heading to the gym and office.

And finally, a medium-sized way I can further model Alexander's behavior in the next month: work overtime to wrap up this manuscript (*Achievement*) so we can remain on schedule for a summer release.

CHAPTER NINE

Excuses or Progress: Choose One

"He that is good for making excuses is seldom good for anything else."
—Benjamin Franklin

ne day, we say, we're going to live a beautiful life. The best life.

We're going to wake up at the best time every morning, do the best workouts, eat the best foods, and do the best things with the best people.

One day, we say, we're going to lose that belly fat, learn that instrument, get that corner office, write that poem about the goat that shagged the pumpkin.

The kicker, though, is that day will never come, because it's always tomorrow, next week, next year, next lifetime. There are always excuses why *today* isn't that day.

Whenever we say, "I would do X, but I can't because Y," it's almost always bullshit, unless Y is "I don't really want to."

That's what most everything in life really comes down to: necessity. There's probably very little we're actually incapable of; there's only our sense of urgency and willingness to act. When we lie to ourselves and say otherwise, what we're really saying is that we find alibis more attractive than achievements, excuses more seductive than excellence, and comfort more desirable than challenge.

We do this because excuses are tempting. They promise freedom from pain, embarrassment, and failure. They lull us into letting ourselves off the hook. Without excuses, we have to face the things we don't want to face and do the things we don't want to do. We have to walk the firing line every day and prove that we're still worthy of our stations. Without excuses, having done and been is never enough. We have to keep doing and becoming.

The world loves to offer us excuses, too. People can't wait to justify our shortcomings and shortfalls for us and thereby attempt to absolve themselves of their own as well. In extreme cases, this can take the form of global excuses that provide cover for any and all failures in life.

According to Dr. Charles R. Snyder, a pioneer in the field of positive psychology, this style of "self-handicapping" can take many forms, ranging from general refrains like "I've had a hard life" to specific ones like a baseball pitcher who complains of a sore arm before a game to protect himself if he performs poorly, as well as set himself up for additional praise if he pitches well despite the nagging arm.[1]

Psychological handicaps and symptoms, such as certain anxieties and phobias, can work as general excuses for flopping as well. "Some people," Dr. Snyder said in a 1984 interview with the *New York Times*, "use problems like test anxiety, shyness or even hypochondriacal disease symptoms as excuses to avoid situations where they fear failure. Self-handicapping can offer an all-purpose out."[1]

We all understand this to some degree. We've all given into excuses to escape realities we didn't want to face. This is a dangerous game to play. Like the lotus fruit of Homer's *Odyssey*, excuses have a narcotic effect, comforting us while warping our sense of reality and sapping us of our spirit and desires. When taken to an extreme, excuse making produces people who actively orchestrate their lives to conform to their pretenses.

Scientifically speaking, the more you make excuses, the more you lose your sense of what psychologists call an "internal locus of control." This is characterized by holding ourselves accountable for both our successes and failures, rather than assigning responsibility mostly (or solely) to factors outside our influence (an "external" locus of control).

For example, an athlete with a strong internal locus of control will credit his success more to hard work rather than innate talent, and an entrepreneur with an internal locus of control will be more likely to chalk a failed venture up to his faulty work rather than bad luck.

Psychologists have been studying locus of control since the 1950s, and they've found that an internal locus of control is associated with greater academic success, higher self-motivation and social maturity, lower incidences of stress and depression, and longer life span.[2]

Scientists have observed that people with an internal locus of control tend to make more money, have more friends, fare better in marriage, and experience more professional success and satisfaction. Those with an external locus of control, however, generally encounter more stress and hardship.

What it comes down to is this: when we refuse to believe that it's okay to give up, to take the easy road out, to look for reasons to be weak, to curse someone or something else for our circumstances, we tap into something primeval that sets extraordinary people apart from everyone else.

Imagine for a moment that you're an eleven-year-old boy with a dream of graduating high school. A boy who lives in the backlands of war-torn Uganda, whose entire family succumbed to disease by the time you were six, and whose grandmother can't afford your school's tuition fee of $43 per month. What do you do? How do you survive, let alone flourish?

That was once reality for James Kassaga Arinaitwe, who refused to abandon his goal of getting a good education and resign himself to working the fields filled with everyone he knew. Instead, he came up with a plan: sell a goat to get shoes, clothes, and a bus ticket to his aunt, who lived near the Ugandan president's country home, and then infiltrate the compound, sneak past the guards, and humbly ask the premier for his assistance.

That's exactly what he did, and it worked. Today, Arinaitwe has two master's degrees, and is the CEO and cofounder of Teach For Uganda, which works to expand educational opportunity to all children in his home country.

Imagine for a moment you've been arrested for writing derogatorily about your government and shipped off to serve an eight-year sentence in forced labor camps with an average life expectancy of one winter. What do you do? How might you view your fate?

Well, you're now Aleksandr Solzhenitsyn, a decorated Soviet soldier who fought against Nazi Germany. In February 1945, while serving in East Prussia, he was arrested by SMERSH for criticizing how Stalin was conducting the war in a private letter written to a friend. In July of the same year, he was convicted in absentia of anti-Soviet propaganda and "founding a hostile organization," and sent to the Gulag.

After spending some time in the camps and witnessing firsthand the pure horrors of communist totalitarianism,

Aleksandr began to reflect on how exactly he had gotten there. Whose fault was it? Whom should he blame? Hitler? Stalin? God?

He came to a different conclusion: it was his fault, because, ultimately, he was playing the same game. He had completely forfeited his relationship with the truth. He had pretended not to see his society degenerating into a brutal monocracy, and even worse, he had fought to advance his captors' tyranny into the world and turned a blind eye to the brutality of his compatriots, who had looted and executed civilians, gang-raped women and young girls to death, and bombed and strafed refugees.

Here's how he later explained it in his earthshaking 1973 book *The Gulag Archipelago*:

> *There is nothing that so assists the awakening of omniscience within us as insistent thoughts about one's own transgressions, errors, mistakes. After the difficult cycles of such ponderings over many years, whenever I mentioned the heartlessness of our highest-ranking bureaucrats, the cruelty of our executioners, I remember myself in my Captain's shoulder boards and the forward march of my battery through East Prussia, enshrouded in fire, and I say: "So were we any better?*

Aleksandr's insistence on accepting responsibility for the entirety of his condition and refusal to point the finger elsewhere inspired him to write the book in which that passage appears. This book chronicled his years in the slave camps, and he hurled it at the USSR like a harpoon and struck a mortal blow. Aleksandr's masterwork destroyed whatever shred of moral credibility Stalin's regime still had left, accelerating its downfall, and eventually won the Nobel Prize.

People like these have the extraordinary ability to do what they say they're going to do no matter what comes.

As the celebrated fashion designer, screenwriter, and Academy Award–nominated director Tom Ford put it, "I guess I'm just one of these people who, when I decide I'm going to do something, I just do it."

When Ford decided to abandon architecture and pursue a career in fashion, he called the prominent sportswear designer Cathy Hardwick every day for a month to ask for an interview. Finally, Hardwick herself answered, hoping to brush away this gadfly. She listened to Tom's spiel, and asked how soon he could be at her office for a meeting. Two minutes later, he arrived at her door. He was calling from the lobby.

Tom convinced Hardwick to hire him as a design assistant, and two years later, he was tapped by Perry Ellis to design jeans. Then, in 1990, Tom moved to Milan to work for Gucci, and over the course of the next decade, he transformed it from a struggling, outworn leather company with about $230 million in annual sales to a chic powerhouse with over $3 billion in annual revenue.

Tom's ascension and apotheosis is a testament to the simple fact that you have to give yourself wholly to something to achieve anything worth having.

Remember these stories when you're tempted to say "I can't."

I can't get into the gym a few days per week, or I don't really want to?

I can't get up early tomorrow to get my workout done, or I don't really want to?

I can't ditch fast food for home-cooked meals, or I don't really want to?

The influential writer Charles Bukowski minced no words in his expression of this enduring truism:

If you're going to try, go all the way. Otherwise, don't even start.

This could mean losing girlfriends, wives, relatives and maybe even your mind. It could mean not eating for three or four days. It could mean freezing on a park bench. It could mean jail. It could mean derision. It could mean mockery— isolation. Isolation is the gift. All the others are a test of your endurance, of how much you really want to do it.

And, you'll do it, despite rejection and the worst odds. And it will be better than anything else you can imagine.

If you're going to try, go all the way. There is no other feeling like that. You will be alone with the gods, and the nights will flame with fire. You will ride life straight to perfect laughter. It's the only good fight there is.

That's power. That's the big secret to stifling excuses. That's how to do the "impossible."

Recommended Reading
Make Your Bed by William H. McRaven

Do This Now

Write down five instances where you witnessed someone making excuses instead of making progress.

Why were these excuses ultimately invalid? What could they

have done if they had really wanted to? Ask "Why?" as many times as you need to get to the ground truth—the real reason they failed.

For example, let's say someone has failed to stick with their workout routine. Why? They say they struggled to wake up for the early workouts. Why? They say they're "just not a morning person." Why? They like to go to bed late. Why? They watch a lot of TV.

Thus, the real reason they stopped working out is watching TV is more important to them than getting fit.

Now write down five instances where you yourself made excuses instead of making progress.

Why were these excuses ultimately invalid? What could you have done if you had really wanted to? Again, ask "Why?" as many times as you need to get to the real reasons.

CHAPTER TEN

Shut Up and Train

*"Opportunity is missed by most people because it is
dressed in overalls and looks like work."*
—*Thomas Edison*

You there.
Yes.
YOU.
pokes your chest
Shut up and train.

Shhhh. I know. You don't have to tell me.

I've heard the same from hundreds—nay, thousands—of others who are perpetually "planning" on getting fit.

You really want to get into shape. But something about not having time. Or needing more sleep. Or fear or lack of know-how or experience or your middle school PE teacher who forced you to run laps until you puked and made you hate exercise.

I don't care. I'm training. You're not. End of story.

So, seriously. Shut up. Shut. Up. And train.

Yeah, it's hard. Some days, it feels like you're trying to swallow the sun. Like you're trying to walk a 220-pound dog or lift dead elephants. Training requires discipline, effort, and sacrifice. There are no free rides. You have to give something to get something.

But let's face it. Training isn't that hard. It's not mortal combat. It's not quantum physics, or even algebra.

I'm not asking you to pick up a sword and shield and enter the arena, wrestle an alligator, or eat a fried tarantula. Hell, I'm not even asking you to make a fool of yourself in a public place, or scrub the stale piss off a public bathroom floor.

I'm asking you to drag your ass up to a bunch of metal every day, and pick it up and put it down like a savage until your muscles burn and your body aches.

Clank. Boom. Thud. The beautiful chorus of a ritual honoring Mother Nature's most cherished touchstone for all her creations: survival of the fittest. Not the richest. Not the wittiest. Not the kindest. The fittest. Money can't buy strength or discipline. Wit can't thicken your hide. Kindness can't stop the world from running you over.

So shut up and train.

Don't talk about training. Stop reading about it. Don't even read my stuff. It'll be here later—after you've trained. When you've put in the work and paid the admission ticket. You go train. Then you come here. Anything else is just foreplay. Masturbation even. That's not how it works.

I really want to train, but . . .

But what? But bullshit.

Writers write. Salespeople sell. Politicians politick. We train.

Oh you're scared, are you? I understand.

It means ditching the excuses, the self-destructive habits, the self-pity shticks. It means opening yourself up to criticism and disappointment. It means announcing to the world that you've been less than perfect, and have somehow found the nerve to raise your standards.

Trust me. I know. I really do. And I don't give a shit, because I'm not telling you to jump out of a plane without a chute. I'm not trying to feed you gas station sushi. Nobody is lurking in the alleys. Your name isn't written on any bullets.

So train. Right now. Go. Train. Don't make me make you.

What? You don't have the time? Oh, okay. Why didn't you say that in the beginning? You're excused, then.

Get real. Who has the time for half of all the stuff we want to do? I'm sorry that life isn't gift wrapping a chunk of your days so you can train in Zen-like comfort and solitude. Join the club. Face the fact that you're going to die with a long to-do list. Make damn sure "start training" isn't on that list.

Oh, you're afraid of messing it up? Of quitting like all the other losers? Welcome to being human. Nobody wants to face-plant. It might leave a scar. People might hiss at us. We might hiss at ourselves. But everyone stumbles and falls. The strong ones get back up a little wiser. A little less likely to fall again.

Or is it that nobody respects that you want to train? Nothing new there. People love to ridicule what they don't understand. And what they wish they had or could do. So who cares what they think? Disrespect is how you know you're getting somewhere. Forget glamor and glory. They tarnish and fade. Dirt and honor? Now we're cooking. Those are the real treasures.

In the final analysis, you're either training or you're not. And I can't do anything for you if you're not training. I can't make you train. I can't strap your lazy limbs to mine and do it for you. This is on you.

So shut up and train. Stop reading this book and train. Whatever you can do right now. I don't care what it is. Start with one hundred push-ups. Then go run some sprints. Who cares if it's random? If it seems pointless? Sweat it out, and admire every bead your body offers you. And then go in for some more.

Once you're done, stop and be proud. Take that self-doubt and punt it across the room, because you're doing it. You're training. Scream it. No, roar. Go ahead. Like a conqueror.

I SAID ROAR, DAMN IT.

And tomorrow?

The plan starts with shutting up and ends with training. Don't call your friends to see if anyone is going to join you. Don't think about how hard it's going to be. Don't you dare tell yourself you deserve a break.

You deserve to train.

And once you've done it enough, you get to say you're doing it.

Recommended Reading

Bigger Leaner Stronger (men) or **Thinner Leaner Stronger** (women) by yours truly :-)

Do This Now

Do at least one workout before reading another page in the book, even if it's an impromptu bodyweight workout, like this:

- Three sets of push-ups to failure with two minutes of rest between each set
- Three sets of air squats to failure with two minutes of rest between each set
- One hundred burpees in as many sets as it takes

- One hundred jumping jacks in as many sets as it takes, or if you're more of a masochist, run five ten-second sprints outside with one minute of rest between each set

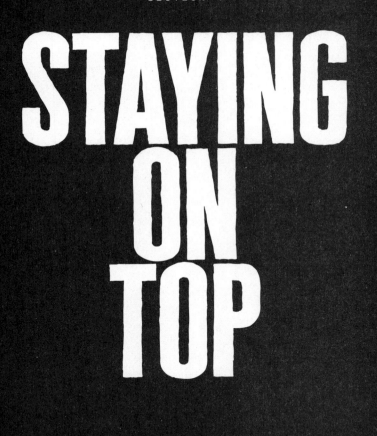

SECTION 4

STAYING ON TOP

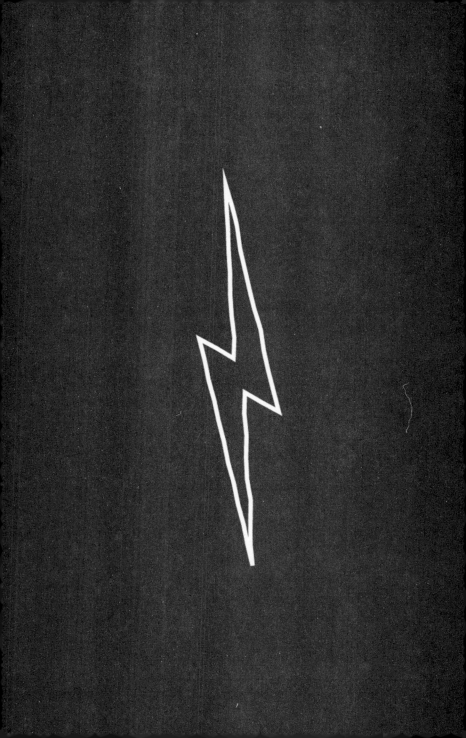

CHAPTER ELEVEN

So, You're Having a Shitty Workout . . .

"Hard choices, easy life. Easy choices, hard life."
—Jerzy Gregorek

You don't want to be in the gym. Everything feels god-awfully heavy. You're just going through the motions, counting down the sets until you can leave. It happens.

I have shitty workouts too, sometimes every week. Sometimes twice per week. Once in a while, I have to slog through a whole run of dreadful sessions, like I've got some kind of low-grade radiation poisoning and every round is just sweaty grunting without aim or purpose.

Why? Sometimes I'm underslept and overworked. Others times I'm nursing an ache or strain. Other times I just can't get into the zone for reasons known best to the Dread Lord Cthulhu.

Again, it happens. The problem is, these days, these freakin' days, I tell you—they really can be suffocating, can't they? Suck the life right out of you.

Well, bad workouts, like bad days at work, home, or the proctologist, are normal. They're just part of the game, the warp and woof of what we do.

In fact, working out is supposed to be hard. That's the point. Easy things are boring things, like shaving our genitals or thumb wrestling. Those are perfectly fine things to do, but they're not going to amount to much. Porno nuts have never helped anyone summit Maslow's pyramid. So don't get it wrong. Working out—and building your best body ever—isn't manscaping. It's not bagging groceries, even though it can feel that way sometimes.

Consider: The act of transforming your body is so much more than merely building muscle or losing fat—it's you *sacrificing who you are for who you want to be*, and then using iron and steel to beat your new form into being. Forging a new you is heat and fire, hammer and anvil, lightning and thunder, not changing your underwear or cutting your nails. It's a mystical, mystifying, and mythological act.

So yeah, sometimes it's hard. Hard as hell. Sometimes you have to leave some blood on the altar. As it should be. As it must be.

Woe is he who believes that things that don't come naturally and easily aren't worth doing, or aren't meant to be done at all. We see this all the time. Person tries something new, person flounders, and person immediately quits in disgrace. Back to binge-watching YouTube vlogs and arguing with strangers on Twitter he goes, because he doesn't get it.

The fact that the thing is hard isn't a sign that it's probably not worth it. The struggle is the point. The struggle is how it signals its worth. The fact that it's hard isn't a sign that you don't belong in the arena. The struggle is how you prove you're worthy.

The influential Greek philosopher Epictetus wrote about this in his *Discourses*:

> *What would have become of Hercules do you think if there had been no lion, hydra, stag or boar—and no savage criminals to rid the world of? What would he have done in the absence of such challenges?*

> *Obviously he would have just rolled over in bed and gone back to sleep. So by snoring his life away in luxury and comfort he never would have developed into the mighty Hercules.*

> *And even if he had, what good would it have done him? What would have been the use of those arms, that physique, and that noble soul, without crises or conditions to stir him into action?*

The message of this allegory extends far beyond classical tales. It strikes at a fundamental aspect of human nature: we can only be as great as our circumstances demand.

Kublai Khan, grandson of Genghis Khan and one of the last great Mongolian rulers, knew this well. Soft lands make soft people, so every year, he would make his soldiers split their time between the decadence of their newly acquired Chinese territories and the austerity of the rugged plains of their homeland, the Steppes. He even kept a plot of grass from his native soil in the garden of his Chinese palace as a personal reminder of the spirit that built his empire.

Rome's eventual rise to prominence started with an inauspicious string of humiliating military defeats that would have broken a weaker state. The early Romans may not have known warfare, but few peoples in history have known how to embrace the struggle better than they. This is what enabled them to cultivate military and diplomatic prowess that would ultimately win them millions of acres of territory stretching from the Atlantic Ocean to the Euphrates, from Britain to Egypt.

Every one of us playing the personal transformation game struggles too. It's hard for me just as it's hard for you and has been hard for everyone who has ever lived. It takes work. Unconscionable amounts of unholy, and sometimes unbearable, work. The work that most people don't want to do. The hard things, the uncomfortable things, the complicated things, the unexciting things, the exhausting things. All the things that never get easier or even enjoyable but must be done regardless.

Building the body of your dreams isn't hard in the same way other work is hard, though. You're not slapping wolverines or wrestling porcupines. When you look at it that way, it's actually pretty easy. But it's also hard, and that's okay. We shouldn't discount what it takes and what it means. It takes resilience. It takes sacrifice. It takes the courage to stop caring so much about things that aren't careworthy.

Remember this when you're having a bad day in the gym, a harder-than-hell workout.

Remember too that sometimes the hardest work moves the needle the most. Sometimes it's on these days that you break through. You never know. So don't let that stop you. Just put your head down, and charge again into the breach.

And remember that no obstacles in your journey are too towering or thorny unless you say they are. There's nothing that can't be overcome with enough perseverance.

"Nothing in the world can take the place of persistence," wrote President Calvin Coolidge. "Talent will not; nothing is more common than unsuccessful men with talent. Genius will not; unrewarded genius is almost a proverb. Education will not; the world is full of educated derelicts. Persistence and determination alone are omnipotent. The slogan 'Press On' has solved and always will solve the problems of the human race."

So, when you're having a hard day, train anyway. Do it because it's hard.

Don't let one bad day rob you of the days that will follow. Days that might be hard too. Harder, even. Who knows. Who cares. It's supposed to be difficult. You're smithing a new body, a new mindset, a new identity. Why should that be easy?

It is what it is. It is what it must be.

Recommended Reading
Meditations by Marcus Aurelius and translated by Gregory Hays

Do This Now

In their fantastic 2017 book *Peak Performance*, Brad Stulberg and Steve Magness wrote about how elite athletes use positive self-talk to improve performance and grit.

"There is widespread evidence that self-talk boosts performance," they wrote. "In particular, studies show that self-talk increases motivation and willingness to endure uncomfortable situations. Self-talk is most effective when what we tell ourselves is short, specific, and, most important, consistent."

For example, when elite runners start feeling pain and discomfort in their workouts (which they all do), they respond differently from most people. Instead of thinking about how painful it is and how much worse it's going to get, or trying to force their way through or fight against it, they have a calm conversation with themselves that goes something like this:

"This is starting to hurt now. It should. I'm running hard.

But I am separate from this pain. It's going to be okay."

In other words, they decide how to respond to the stress of the workout, and it makes all the difference in their mindset (they relax) and performance (they put up better times).

Similarly, a basketball player who's nervous at the free throw line might tell himself, "I've done this before. I can make this shot." A public speaker might calm his nerves by saying, "Everyone out there is like me—awkward and vulnerable." A runner who has fallen behind might remind herself, "Anything can happen. I'm not out of this. Don't let up."

Even better is self-talk that includes the element of purpose—of why you're pushing past the pain and disappointment.

"Regardless of what you are doing—whether you are using your body, mind, or soul—repeating a purpose-driven mantra during times of fear, pain, or apprehension can yield big benefits," Stulberg and Magness explain. "Doing so grounds us, attenuates negative emotions, and quiets our ego."

Here are a few examples they give of this:

- A professional bike racer who wrote the following mantra and stuck it on his handlebars so he sees it whenever the pace, and pain, picks up and he puts his head down: *To inspire other people to get out of their comfort zones and live life to its fullest.*
- A middle manager at a health care company who reminds herself why she fields inane and frustrating questions from frontline staff: *To make a difference in the lives of other human beings.*
- An artist who finds inspiration to do the boring non-art stuff to fulfill her purpose: *To create beautiful art that moves people.*

This works equally well for all kinds of stress, whether physical, mental, or emotional. Instead of groaning to ourselves, we can choose to respond differently, with something short, specific, and inspiring, and leaven both our perception of the circumstances we're facing and our ability to deal with them effectively.

Now it's your turn.

Revisit the purposes you wrote down at the end of Chapter 1, and the final one in particular.

If it's lengthy, condense it down to a simple, one-sentence statement that captures its most compelling elements.

This is now your fitness mantra, and you should come back to it whenever the seas get choppy and you're slogging through workouts, or debating even showing up.

To make sure you always have your mantra accessible, write it down, cut it out, and keep it on you at all times (in your wallet, for instance), or save it digitally in software you can access on your phone, like Evernote or Google Drive.

CHAPTER TWELVE

The Curse of Complaining

"Be less concerned with what you have than with what you are."
—Socrates

Think about your last couple of days.

How many times did you hear someone complain about something? Maybe it was a moan about something petty, like the weather, or a groan about something personal, like the holiday weight that they still haven't lost, or a gripe about something more significant, like the economy or political circus.

My guess is you can recall dozens if not scores of conversations, comments, emails, texts, and tweets that involved—if not revolved around—complaining. Maybe you even joined in yourself.

For many people, grumbling isn't an exception; it's a way of life. They're obsessed with what's wrong, and they'll vent about anything and everything to anyone who will listen.

It's Monday again. A guy is curling in the squat rack again. They still don't make enough money. The free coffee shop WiFi is always too slow. It's colder than it should be in January. Their friend's Facebook status updates have typos. Someone left the toilet seat up.

Why devote so much time and energy to whining, when it's scientifically proven to increase stress and anxiety, sour mood, lead to more negative thinking, and hamper progress toward solutions and goals?[1]

Why do it, when one-tenth of that time and energy put into finding solutions would dramatically improve conditions for the better?

Some people prefer being a victim. They're hooked on how it arouses sympathy, lowers expectations, excuses negativity, and relieves the burden of personal responsibility. By putting their difficulties on display, they hope to convince people to judge them more leniently for their shortcomings and failures and praise them more enthusiastically for their successes.

Sigmund Freud once commented on this, writing that "neurotics complain of their illness, but they make the most of it, and when it comes to taking it away from them they will defend it like a lioness her young."

Don't be one of these people. Underlying all their grievances is the ugly reality that they're just managing their lives poorly.

"Everything that happens is either endurable or not," wrote the legendary Roman emperor and stoic philosopher Marcus Aurelius. "If it's endurable, then endure it. Stop complaining. If it's unendurable, then stop complaining. Your destruction will mean its end as well. Just remember: you can endure anything your mind can make endurable, by treating it as in your interest to do so. In your interest, or in your nature."

Don't go looking for sympathy. Most people don't care about your problems, and many are secretly glad that you have them. Don't compromise your standards. No matter what you want to do, moderation won't get you very far. Nothing succeeds like excess. Don't shirk your duties. The more you suffer voluntarily, the less you'll suffer involuntarily.

And whatever you do, don't whinge. If you don't like something, do something to change it. Don't complain; just work harder. And if you ultimately can't change it—no matter how undeserved or unreasonable it is—then change your mind about it, because that's something you can always control. To quote Aurelius again, "Choose not to be harmed, and you won't feel harmed. Don't feel harmed, and you haven't been."

Don't think you can't do this, either. No matter how challenging a situation might be, you can respond to it in one of two ways: you can view it as a challenge or a threat, and that choice can make all the difference in how it affects you.

To quote Brad Stulberg and Steve Magness again in *Peak Performance*:

> *Some individuals learn to assess stressors as challenges rather than threats. This outlook, which researchers call a "challenge response," is characterized by viewing stress as something productive, and, much like we've written, as a stimulus for growth. In the midst of stress, those who demonstrate a challenge response proactively focus on what they can control. With this outlook, negative emotions like fear and anxiety decrease. This response better enables these individuals to manage and even thrive under stress.*

Reframing stress as a constructive rather than destructive force is more powerful than you might think. It not only positively influences your attitudes and feelings; it also impacts your physiology.

Studies show that people who react to stress with a "challenge response" release more DHEA than those who don't, which counteracts the negative effects of cortisol, and can even confer health benefits.[2]

This helps explain why research conducted by scientists at the University of Wisconsin found that people who view stress positively have a 43 percent lower chance of premature death than those who view it negatively.[3]

One way of doing this is choosing to view feelings of anxiety, stress, and fear that accompany uncomfortable situations as natural responses that can be redirected toward positive outcomes.

This is one of the many "little" things that sets elite athletes apart from amateur ones—the top-tier competitors embrace pre-event nerves as feelings of excitement, as opposed to fighting them in an attempt to "calm down."[4]

We can use the same strategy to better cope with any situation or event that produces similar feelings in us. As much as some mistakes and missteps can hurt, they're also precious opportunities to learn lessons that may otherwise never come to light.

In fact, you can even view the process of pushing through and reflecting on pain and figuring out the lesson to be learned as a game of sorts, and the better you get at it, the more you'll come to enjoy your struggles and the rewards they provide.

"I have found it helpful to think of my life as if it were a game in which each problem I face is a puzzle I need to solve," Ray Dalio shared in *Principles*. "By solving the puzzle, I get a gem in the form of a principle that helps me avoid the same sort of problem in the future. Collecting these gems continually improves my decision making, so I am able to ascend to higher and higher levels of play in which the game gets harder and the stakes become ever greater."

Don't underestimate how much struggle you can endure, either. You're not as fragile as you might think, and you can push yourself much further than you probably realize.

That's what the founder of Marquis Jets, Jesse Itzler, learned after spending a month with a 230-pound retired Navy SEAL named David Goggins, which Itzler chronicled in his rollicking 2015 book *Living with a SEAL*.

The two men met at a hundred-mile ultramarathon, which Jesse ran with five of his friends as a relay race, with a tent, team of masseuses, and smorgasbord of food in tow. David brought a folding chair, bottle of water, and bag of crackers, and he ran it alone. By mile seventy, David's ankles were the size of grapefruits; he had broken all the small bones in his feet and was suffering from kidney damage, but he just kept going.

Jesse couldn't believe what he had witnessed. Weeks later, he decided to track down David's contact information and call to ask how he was able to do something that Jesse, an experienced endurance athlete, had previously thought impossible.

By the end of the call, Jesse wanted to meet David in person. By the end of that first meeting, Jesse was so impressed with the man's character and approach to living that he asked him to come and live with his family for a month to help him break out of his stultifying routine, whip him into better shape, and hopefully teach him some lessons that would help him do even better in his life.

On the day David arrived, he asked Jesse to show him how many pull-ups he could do. Jesse did eight, barely. David told him to go again, and he eked out six. One more time, the former SEAL said, and Jesse fought to get three or four before his arms gave out. "That's it," he said. "I can't do any more." David smirked. "We're not leaving here until you've done one hundred more." Jesse's eyes widened. *We're going to be here for a long time*, he thought. And he was right—it took several hours—but he did it, one pull-up at a time.

The point?

"Whenever you think you're done and entirely ready to give

out," David told Jesse, "you're only 40 percent of the way there."

Over the course of the next thirty days, Jesse would learn that this "40 percent rule" applies to a lot more than pull-ups, and that he could endure far more discomfort than he'd ever experienced before.

The same goes for all of us. No matter how physically, mentally, or emotionally grueling a situation might be, and no matter how much we might want to throw in the towel, we still have a lot more to give. We can push ourselves a lot further and triumph over far more difficulty than we give ourselves credit for.

Several years ago, I received an email from a man named Robert who had just finished reading my book *Bigger Leaner Stronger*. He was a fifty-two-year-old overachieving CEO who worked seventy to eighty hours per week. He was overweight and out of shape, and popping pills every day to cope with back, knee, and shoulder pain. His cholesterol, triglycerides, and blood pressure were too high, and his doctor was concerned that his body could only take so much abuse before seizing up.

Robert was writing because he was fairly certain that the diet and exercise advice provided in my book wasn't going to work for him. He didn't see a way out of the ditch he had dug for himself.

I had worked with many Roberts before, so I reassured him that everything in the book was going to work just as well for him as it did the college kids. I helped him create a diet plan he could actually follow and a minimalistic workout routine that fit his busy schedule (and that his doctor approved of).

He struggled at first. He struggled to do his butt-crack-of-dawn workouts. He struggled to make time to eat well. He struggled to moderate his sugar and junk food intake. Every week, though, he would email me on his progress. Every week, his waist got a little smaller, his lifts got a little better, and his cravings got a little weaker. Every week, he felt a little more focused, encouraged, and determined.

Just three months after starting my program, his doctor couldn't believe what she was witnessing. Robert had lost twenty-four pounds and gained a considerable amount of muscle, his joint pains had all but vanished, and his blood work had done a one-eighty. Robert would go on to see his abs for the first time in his life, reduce his risk of heart disease by triple digits, and help his children develop the same healthy habits that were changing his life.

So remember: the more someone deals in complaints, the more they're telegraphing their weakness of character and inability to act. They sit on the sidelines and do the only thing they're capable of: carping and criticizing those who are in the arena, struggling and striving.

Don't be one of them. Refuse to complain.

Recommended Reading
A Complaint Free World by Will Bowen

Do This Now

A simple way to inoculate ourselves against unproductive complaining is the "21-day no-complaint challenge" outlined in the 2013 book *A Complaint Free World* by Will Bowen.

The challenge is simple: you win by going twenty-one days without complaining, and to keep it top of mind, you wear a rubber bracelet on one of your wrists. (A rubber band works just fine if you don't want to buy one of his.)

If you complain, you switch the band to the other wrist and restart your day count at zero.

According to Will, you should switch wrists whenever you "gossip, criticize, or complain," but without precise definitions and guardrails, these concepts are open to interpretation. And so I propose this: you switch when you voice a negative description of a person or event with no indication as to how the problem could be fixed.

Therefore, these types of statements would require a wrist switch:

- "I can't believe I had to wait an hour for my lunch today. What a waste of time."
- "Johnny can be such an ass."
- "This WiFi sucks."

And these wouldn't:

- "I waited an hour for my lunch today. Next time, I'm going earlier to beat the crowd."
- "Johnny is being an ass about this project. I'm going to communicate directly with his superior and get her agreement, and then he'll be out of the way."
- "This WiFi sucks. I'm going to tether to my phone instead."

Will also considers telling someone else they're complaining a flunk, but I disagree. I'm a big believer in both giving and receiving constructive criticism.

If you find this challenge difficult at first, I understand. I thought I would pass with flying colors on my first attempt, but didn't make it more than a few days before having to restart. Eventually, a few months later, I made it through. It also made me painfully aware of how much time people spend grousing about things they can't or won't do anything about, and how easily I used to join into such conversations, even if just to fire off a few rounds of flak.

Stick with the challenge for as long as it takes to pass, and I think you'll be pleasantly surprised at how much of an impact changing your thoughts and words can have on your life. You'll start viewing your problems more practically, you'll get better at ignoring petty frustrations and negativity, and you'll become less inclined to complain even to yourself about undesirable situations or conditions you face.

CHAPTER THIRTEEN

The Positivity Paradox

"You can't stop the waves, but you can learn to surf."
—Jon Kabat-Zinn

As the highest-ranking officer in the "Hanoi Hilton" prisoner-of-war camp during the height of the Vietnam War, Jim Stockdale knew he wasn't getting out anytime soon.

He was tortured regularly, and had no prisoner's rights, release date, or, it would seem, reason to believe he would live long enough to see his family or country again.

Despite all this, Stockdale refused to give in. He did everything he could to help his fellow prisoners survive the ordeal and to stymie his captors' attempts at using him and his comrades for propaganda, even going as far as disfiguring himself so he couldn't be held up as an example of a "well-treated prisoner."

He encoded intelligence messages into his letters to his wife, risking brutal punishment and death, devised guidelines for dealing with torture that increased his fellow soldiers' odds of survival, created a Morse code-like system of communication using taps to ease isolation anxiety among the men, and more.

In the end, Jim Stockdale spent eight years in captivity, and after his release following the American withdrawal from the war, he was awarded the Congressional Medal of Honor.

It's hard to imagine, even for a moment, what Stockdale's experience must have been like. How in the hell did he not collapse into a completely catatonic state? How did he find the strength to stand up every day and continue working against the enemy? What inspired his unbreakable will?

"I never lost faith in the end of the story," he later said. "I never doubted not only that I would get out, but also that I would prevail in the end and turn the experience into the defining event of my life, which, in retrospect, I would not trade."

If we were to leave Stockdale's story at that, we could chalk up his resilience to the power of positive thinking and optimism. But when he was asked who didn't make it, his reply was surprising.

"The optimists," he said. "Oh, they were the ones who said, 'We're going to be out by Christmas.' And Christmas would come, and Christmas would go. Then they'd say, 'We're going to be out by Easter.' And Easter would come, and Easter would go. And then Thanksgiving, and then it would be Christmas again. And they died of a broken heart.

"This is a very important lesson," he added. "You must never confuse faith that you will prevail in the end—which you can never afford to lose—with the discipline to confront the most brutal facts of your current reality, whatever they might be."

In other words, hope is vital, but unbridled optimism, bordering on delusion, can be self-defeating and even dangerous.

Winston Churchill knew this as well, which is why he created the Statistical Office early in the war, and assigned it a very specific job: to feed him unfiltered facts and data about the conflict, no matter how disturbing.

"I . . . had no need for cheering dreams," he wrote as the Nazi blitzkrieg was stampeding through Europe. "Facts are better than dreams." Churchill relied heavily on this department throughout the entire war, and couldn't have made the decisions he made without the willingness to face things as they were, not as he wished they were.

Both of these men understood the importance of embracing optimism without giving themselves over completely to *optimism bias*—the belief that we're less likely to suffer from misfortune and more likely to attain success than reality would suggest.

As Daniel Kahneman explains in *Thinking, Fast and Slow*, "Most of us view the world as more benign than it really is, our own attributes as more favorable than they truly are, and the goals we adopt as more achievable than they are likely to be. We also tend to exaggerate our ability to forecast the future, which fosters optimistic overconfidence."

In other words, most of us (up to 80 percent, according to most estimates) generally view ourselves as statistical outliers, and this is why so many people tend to grossly discount their chances of getting divorced, being in a car accident, or developing a serious disease, and greatly overestimate their chances of getting a job out of college (and the amount of money they'll be paid for it), their ability to make an accurate clinical diagnosis, and how long they will live.[1]

Ironically, the most optimistically biased among us are also the most likely to smoke, have unsafe sex, forgo medical screenings, seat belts, and insurance, and overspend, while those who are more pessimistically inclined are more likely to succeed in business and lose less money while gambling, and tend to make terrific lawyers.[2]

On the other hand, we also know that optimism and positivity can pay significant dividends. Our lives are deeply influenced by optimistic individuals. These are the inventors, entrepreneurs, and social leaders who seek king-sized challenges, take daunting risks, and remain resilient in the face of stupefying setbacks.

To quote Kahneman again, "Optimists are normally cheerful and happy, and therefore popular; they are resilient in adapting to failures and hardships, their chances of clinical depression are reduced, their immune system is stronger, they take better care of their health, they feel healthier than others and are in fact likely to live longer. A study of people who exaggerate their expected life span beyond actuarial predictions showed that they work longer hours, are more optimistic about their future income, are more likely to remarry after divorce (the classic 'triumph of hope over experience'), and are more prone to bet on individual stocks."

We also know that a heavy dose of pessimism isn't the antidote to optimism bias. Professor and happiness expert Martin Seligman explained it like this: "Research has revealed, predictably, that pessimism is maladaptive in most endeavors: Pessimistic life insurance agents make fewer sales attempts, are less productive and persistent, and quit more readily than optimistic agents. Pessimistic undergraduates get lower grades, relative to their SATs and past academic record, than optimistic students..."[3]

Instead, we need to cultivate a mindset that is mildly biased toward optimism, not blinded by it. We want to be someone who "punches up the positive" without losing track of reality, even when we don't like what it presents us.

We're going to suffer misfortunes and disappointments, people are going to let us down, and we're going to let ourselves down, and no matter how disheartening any of these events will be, we must be able to acknowledge them while also maintaining the belief that we will prevail in the end.

Beware the Great Western Disease

Most people assume that their general circumstances mostly determine how they feel about their lives, and that the small-scale day-to-day details matter far less than the large-scale outcomes.

Two decades of scientific research into happiness and positivity have painted a different picture. They have confirmed things most of us would assume to be true—on the whole, the affluent are happier than the poor, those in good romantic relationships are happier than those who aren't, healthy people are happier than sick people, and those who participate in their churches are happier than those who don't—but it has also shown that while the big wins and losses in our lives do make us happier and sadder, they don't have as much impact as we think they will.

Instead, what we choose to focus on, how we internalize failures and difficulties, and how often we experience and acknowledge positive emotions, even if fleeting, are far more predictive of our long-term happiness.

According to Daniel Gilbert, Harvard psychology professor, and author of the top-selling 2006 book *Stumbling on Happiness*, very few experiences affect us for more than a few months or so.

"When good things happen, we celebrate for a while and then sober up," he said in a 2012 interview with *Harvard Business Review*. "When bad things happen, we weep and whine for a while and then pick ourselves up and get on with it."[4]

Six years ago, my income was a fraction of what it is now, and I had tens of thousands of dollars of credit card debt (the backwash of my early twenties, which involved a lot of gallivanting around Europe).

I truly believed that multiplying my earnings, eliminating debt, and building significant savings and investments was going to fill me with radiant joy. It hasn't. It has eliminated financial worries, but on the whole, my experience has been more or less in line with research conducted by Daniel Kahneman that found that once you've achieved a certain level of income, further earnings can continue to impact how satisfied you are with yourself and where your life is going, but not how much pleasure you derive from your everyday living.[5]

In other words, there's a point where making more money might make you feel better about yourself in the abstract, but won't do much for your daily mood. Kahneman concluded that this number is $75,000 per year, but this one-size-fits-all prescription fails to take into account objective factors like cost of living, number of dependents, and inflation, as well as subjective ones like goals and purposes.

For instance, $75,000 per year goes a lot further for a single guy living in Meridian, Mississippi, in 2009 and working contentedly as a corporate clerk than a married couple with three children living in Manhattan in 2017 and bootstrapping their startup.

Nevertheless, Kahneman's basic assertion rings true: money reaches the point of diminishing emotional returns a lot faster than most of us realize.

A telling example of this can be found in a study conducted by scientists from Northwestern University and the University of Massachusetts. They asked recent winners of the Illinois State Lottery, and recent victims of horrible accidents who were now paraplegic or quadriplegic, about happiness in their lives.[6]

In interviews with the scientists, participants were asked to rate how much pleasure they got from everyday activities like chatting with friends, watching TV, eating breakfast, laughing at jokes, and receiving compliments. After the data was analyzed, the scientists were surprised to learn that while the winners reported more present happiness than the victims, the victims weren't nearly as unhappy as was expected, and rated their daily routine experiences more positively than the lottery winners.

This is due at least in part to what is known as the hedonic treadmill or hedonic adaptation, which is the tendency to get used to whatever makes us acutely happier. Here's how the authors of the study explained it:

> *Eventually, the thrill of winning the lottery will itself wear off. If all things are judged by the extent to which they depart from a baseline of past experience, gradually even the most positive events will cease to have impact as they themselves are absorbed into the new baseline against which further events are judged. Thus, as lottery winners become accustomed to the additional pleasures made possible by their new wealth, these pleasures should be experienced as less intense and should no longer contribute very much to their general level of happiness.*

In other words, new lovers, jobs, and toys are exhilarating, until they're not.

As most of us think these are the types of things that will ultimately make us happy, we can also infer that we humans are generally awful at predicting what will put a smile on our faces every day.

That's exactly what research conducted by scientists at Harvard University and the University of Virginia has confirmed: most people are shockingly bad at predicting how they will feel in the future, how intensely they will feel that way, and how long the feelings will last, and especially when money is involved.[7]

For example, studies show that a shorter commute is more likely to brighten your days than a significant pay raise, receiving a paid vacation is more likely to raise your spirits than a wad of cash, and having more free time is probably more conducive to your well-being than making more money, but which of those options has more immediate appeal to you? The money, or the commute, vacation, or free time?[8]

This bias is at the heart of the Great Western Disease—the idea that we'll finally be happy when we buy that house, or get that six-pack, partner, job, or raise. We won't.

Here's how the father-and-son duo Robert Biswas-Diener and Ed Diener put it in their 2009 book *Happiness*:

> It is just so tempting for myself, for everyone, to think about happiness as something that happens on the other side of the finish line. "If I marry the right person, I get the right commute, I get the right job, I get that paycheck, I go on that vacation, I'm going to end up feeling happy." Happiness is a whole lot more like a roller coaster, with ups and downs that just continues and continues and continues. I can guarantee you that in your future, you will have moments of happiness and moments of unhappiness. Happiness, because it is a process that happens sometimes throughout the day and across the week and over the course of months; it's something that needs to be managed on an ongoing basis.

As you can imagine, that process is multiplex, and our understanding of it is evolving, but scientists have isolated a handful of ways to increase our happiness quotient.

What You See Is What You Get

In her 2009 book *Rapt*, science writer Winifred Gallagher proposed a "grand unified theory" of the mind:

*Like fingers pointing to the moon, other diverse disciplines
from anthropology to education, behavioral economics
to family counseling, similarly suggest that the skillful
management of attention is the sine qua non of the good
life and the key to improving virtually every aspect of your
experience.*

She concluded this after an unexpected and terrifying cancer diagnosis that led her on a five-year odyssey into the realm of positive psychology, and it upends how most of us think about how we experience our lives.

In short, decades of research has demonstrated that we construct our worldview based on *what we pay attention to*, not what *is*. As Gallagher puts it: "Who you are, what you think, feel, and do, what you love—is the sum of what you focus on."

An amusing but illustrative example of how much truth this statement holds is what has come to be known as the Tetris Effect.

Tetris, as you probably know, is a simple game that involves rotating and moving falling shapes so they form unbroken lines. Play enough of this game, and you'll notice a rather disconcerting shift in how you think, dream, and even perceive the world around you.

That's what scientists at Harvard Medical School found when they had twenty-seven people play many hours of Tetris for three consecutive days. For several days after the study, some participants couldn't stop seeing shapes everywhere they went, and others dreamt every night of shapes falling from the sky.[9]

One Tetris addict (yes, they're out there) wrote in the *Philadelphia City Paper* that when he shops for cereal, he notices how perfectly the boxes could fit together to make unbroken rows, when he goes for a run, he imagines rearranging the bricks in walls to create even lines, and when he gazes at the skyline, he ponders how he could flip buildings to fill gaps in the vista.[10]

What's the deal? Is there something about Tetris that somehow loosens our grip on reality? Not quite.

The Tetris Effect is a normal physical process that occurs in the brain when certain cognitive patterns are repeated over and over, and it extends far beyond video games. The more we repeat any pattern of thinking or behaving, the more likely we are to exhibit it generally.

As Shawn Achor described in his 2010 book *The Happiness Advantage*, this is why tax auditors, who spend inordinate amounts of time scanning forms for errors, can begin to approach their entire lives like an audit, noting only faults in work performance reviews and subpar grades on their kids' report cards, and why many lawyers admit to the habits of "deposing" their children at the dinner table every day and mentally tallying how many billable hours they're forfeiting when they're spending time with their spouses.

The psychological stickiness of patterns isn't inherently bad, but when we can't "unstick" ourselves and turn them on and off at will, we become more susceptible to stress, depression, health problems, and even substance abuse.

Fortunately, overriding ingrained ways of thinking and acting can be as simple as consciously managing our attention and regularly directing it toward the positive.

To fully appreciate this, let's do a personal experiment. Take a moment to observe your physical surroundings, and for the next several minutes, look around and ask yourself a few questions, paying attention to how it impacts your mood: *What's right about this environment? What am I okay with? What can I enjoy, admire, and even celebrate?*

As you'll see, it doesn't take much of this before your heart begins to warm.

Bask in the good vibes you've created for a minute, and then, see what happens when you do the opposite. This time, look around and find what's wrong with your current environment, what bothers you, and what should be improved (and if you want to spoil the fun even faster, consider who's likely to blame for all of it).

Notice how quickly the glow fades?

Objectively speaking, nothing has changed between these exercises. You're still occupying the same space and surveying the same environment, which still contains things that can be seen as both wonderful and woeful. How you feel about these realities, though, is determined by your frame of mind. Choose to see the good, and you will feel good; choose to see the bad, and you will feel bad.

In this way, we have a surprising amount of control over our emotions, and can "turn on" positivity almost whenever we want by simply controlling our attention.

This is particularly relevant to us fitness folk, because of how easy it is to compare ourselves to others and see only the things we don't like about our bodies. Don't think that gaining a certain amount of muscle or achieving a certain body fat percentage will change that, either. No matter how good you might look, there's always someone just a tap away on Instagram who looks better, and the more we direct our attention to our inadequacies, the more dissatisfied we'll be with what we see in the mirror.

This is a slippery slope that leads to the unhealthy extremes of fitness—body dysmorphia, eating disorders, excessive exercising, and so on—and an easy way to avoid it is to regularly direct our attention to what we like about our bodies instead.

In fact, why not start right now? What's good about your

body? What can you admire? What's going right?

Answer those questions every day, and you might be surprised how much it boosts your mood, confidence, and sense of well-being.

The Story of Your Life

Recall something that got you down recently. A fight with your partner, junk food binge, work or life disruption, whatever.

Now recall the story you told yourself about this event. How long did you say it would last for? Did you assume it was confined to that specific person, place, or time, or that it was more universal or general in nature? Did you conclude it was entirely your fault, or were external factors in play as well?

The nature of the story you told yourself represents what psychologists would call your "explanatory style," and research conducted by scientists at the University of Michigan shows that it probably falls into one of two buckets—optimistic or pessimistic—and greatly impacts how you view and cope with life in general.[11]

The optimistic view of bad events is characterized by impermanence, particularity, and impersonality, whereas the pessimistic view has the opposite character. In other words, optimists tend to view negative events as temporary ("My boss is probably just having a bad day"), specific to a certain situation ("This diet sucks"), and not entirely their fault ("They just didn't give me a chance"), whereas pessimists see bad things as long-lasting ("My boss is always a bastard"), generalized ("Dieting is useless"), and internally caused ("I'm terrible at interviewing").

Furthermore, these explanatory styles flip for positive events: optimists tend to see good things as permanent ("I always figure out a way to get what I want"), universal ("I'm smart"), and internal ("My skill helped me stand out."), whereas pessimists see them as temporary ("I got lucky this time"), limited ("I'm smart at math"), and external ("My teammates' skill made me look better than I am").

Explanatory styles make for very different lives. A number of studies show that people who usually tell themselves optimistic stories have stronger immune systems, take better care of themselves, find it easier to sustain friendships, and generally encounter fewer negative life events than those whose stories are continually pessimistic. Optimistic athletes, students, and workers tend to outperform pessimistic ones of equal talent, and optimistic stump speeches tend to win more elections than pessimistic ones.[12]

I've helped thousands of men and women lose fat, build muscle, and get healthy, and here's a situation I encounter all too often:

Chris has been following his meal plan and workout regimen for a few weeks now and has made steady improvements. Then, one night after work, he heads out with friends for drinks and winds up eating a few handfuls of the greasy, delicious foods brought to the table.

Immediately afterward, he's upset with himself for "ruining" his diet. Steaming, he berates himself, "Perfect, Chris. There goes this week's progress. I can't believe how weak I am. I can't even hang out with some friends without stuffing my fat face with junk food. How pathetic. You know what? I'm going to eat ice cream when I get home too. That's what a pig would do, right?"

Later that night, Chris gobbles down two containers of Ben & Jerry's Half Baked and plods to bed, disgusted with himself.

It didn't have to go this way. The path from nibbling on nachos and wings at the bar to slurping down pints of ice cream was manufactured by Chris. His story about why he ate the food in the first place ("I'm weak") and his conclusion ("My diet is blown") were highly and unnecessarily pessimistic. If he had rejected his knee-jerk reaction to the snacking and reframed it, the outcome could have been very different.

"Hold on, Chris," he could have said. "I didn't eat *that* much—a few chicken wings and nachos is what, a few hundred calories? My dinner was a bit lighter than usual too. I bet I'll end today only slightly above my caloric target, and if I *really* care, I can eat a bit less or move a bit more tomorrow. Also, eating a little too much today doesn't mean I'm weak. Look at how good I've been over the last few weeks, bringing lunches to work and turning down the cookies, doughnuts, and candies everyone passes around. More importantly, I shouldn't let a minor slip-up turn into a fiasco. That makes no sense. The smart thing to do is chalk the night up to a hiccup, forgive myself, and carry on with the plan."

This is the "secret" to guilt-free dieting and exercising. So long as you can stick to the plan fairly well most of the time and keep calm when you stumble (and you *will* stumble occasionally, because we all do), you'll never struggle to improve your body composition. Things may take a little longer or be a little less straightforward than you'd like, but your wheels will never fall off.

So, the next time you face adversity of any kind, pay attention to your explanatory style, and if it's tainted with pessimism—if the story is permanent, universal, or self-abusive in nature—stop to dispute your assumptions.

Instead of automatically catastrophizing events, argue with yourself to the contrary. Is it really true that this *always* happens? How much does this moment *really* say about the whole? Is that insidiously personal failure the only determining factor, or were there also circumstances outside your control?

You'll find that most of the pessimistic beliefs and assumptions that pop into your head after something bad happens are remarkably easy to unravel. They rarely have much supporting evidence or logic, and they often quickly yield to more optimistic explanations.

Similarly, when good things happen to you, take a moment to celebrate with an optimistic story. What about this win is likely permanent, pervasive, and personal? Have you always had a knack for this kind of thing? Are your opponents just easy to beat? Were you naturally charming? Can you take advantage of lucky situations? Can you count on your skill?

These are the things that positive, uplifting mindsets are made of.

The Power of Productive Pessimism

In the beginning of this chapter, I said that we need to cultivate a mindset that is mildly biased toward optimism, not blinded by it, and that we want to be someone who "punches up the positive" without losing track of reality, even when we don't like what it presents us.

So far, we've discussed how to use optimism to be more productive, effective, resilient, confident, and cheerful, but not how to know when to take off the rose-tinted glasses and grab for a dash of productive pessimism instead.

The first step is understanding that when judiciously applied, pessimism does have its uses. To quote Martin Seligman again in his 2011 book *Learned Optimism*:

> *The company also needs its pessimists, the people who have an accurate knowledge of present realities. They must make sure grim reality continually intrudes upon the optimists.*

> *The treasurer, the CPAs, the financial vice-president, the*
> *business administrators, the safety engineers—all these need*
> *an accurate sense of how much the company can afford, and*
> *of danger. Their role is to caution, their banner is the yellow*
> *flag.*

In the same book, Seligman proposes a simple strategy for exercising pessimism productively, which he calls "flexible optimism." Here's how he explains it:

> *The fundamental guideline for not deploying optimism is to*
> *ask what the cost of failure is in the particular situation. If*
> *the cost of failure is high, optimism is the wrong strategy. The*
> *pilot in the cockpit deciding whether to de-ice the plane one*
> *more time, the partygoer deciding whether to drive home*
> *after drinking, the frustrated spouse deciding whether to start*
> *an affair that, should it come to light, would break up the*
> *marriage should not use optimism. Here the costs of failure*
> *are, respectively, death, an auto accident, and a divorce. Using*
> *techniques that minimize those costs is inappropriate. On the*
> *other hand, if the cost of failure is low, use optimism.*

In other words, when faced with a tricky situation, ask yourself: "What's the cost of being wrong here? What's at stake?" If the potential downsides are significant, then you can save yourself from making crushing mistakes by consciously shifting your mindset toward skepticism and dubiousness, before deploying optimism. If the costs of being wrong are negligible, however, allow yourself to remain optimistic.

Daniel Kahneman echoed this brand of "cautious" optimism in *Thinking, Fast and Slow.* "Optimism is good for staying motivated once you've begun but can be an impediment when analyzing whether you should start in the first place and for planning the endeavor," he wrote.

For example, if you're considering going on a date with that cute guy or gal you met at the gym, there's no need for pessimism. What's the cost of being wrong? A socially awkward evening that will make for a silly story to share with your friends?

If, however, you're considering investing considerable time and money into a new business venture, don't automatically leap into positive arguments and predictions, because even minor misjudgments in the beginning can make for major headaches down the road.

When the stakes are high, it's a good idea to start your analysis with what chief scientist of Klein Associates Gary Klein calls a *premortem.*

"A premortem is the hypothetical opposite of a postmortem," he wrote in a 2007 *Harvard Business Review* article. "A postmortem in a medical setting allows health professionals and the family to learn what caused a patient's death. Everyone benefits except, of course, the patient. A premortem in a business setting comes at the beginning of a project rather than the end, so that the project can be improved rather than autopsied. Unlike a typical critiquing session, in which project team members are asked what might go wrong, the premortem operates on the assumption that the 'patient' has died, and so asks what did go wrong. The team members' task is to generate plausible reasons for the project's failure."[13]

Klein got the idea from a study conducted by scientists at the University of Colorado that found that *prospective hindsight*—imagining that an event has already occurred—can increase the ability to correctly identify reasons for future outcomes by up to 30 percent.[14]

From this paper, Klein devised his premortem procedure and

outlined it in his 2004 book *The Power of Intuition*, and it goes like this:

Start by assuming that the undertaking has failed spectacularly. Then, over the next few minutes, write down every reason you can think of for the failure, and pay special attention to the kinds of things you might not want to consider as potential problems due to ego or, if you're in a group, impoliteness.

Then, revisit your plans in light of the pitfalls you've uncovered, and generate ideas as to how you can minimize their likelihood of occurring or avoid them altogether.

Klein also recommends that you periodically review your premortem list as you make progress on an endeavor and circumstances change, reflecting on new and different ways to fail and their antidotes.

I once went through this exercise with a woman named Maria who wanted to follow my *Thinner Leaner Stronger* program. She was gearing up to embark on a journey to cut her body fat percentage in half, and her reasons for failure included:

- Too many opportunities to overeat due to junk food in the house and socializing.
- Fear of being uncomfortable at the gym and feeling judged by other people.
- An inability to consistently go to bed and wake up on time to do her workouts.
- Peer pressure from friends and family to abandon the goal and accept herself the way she is.

To prevent these things from stopping her, she stopped buying her favorite ice cream and chips; recruited a friend to hit the gym with her to make the experience more inviting; gradually worked her bedtime back as opposed to suddenly changing it by a couple of hours and started placing her alarm clock across the room; ate something before going to social events; and spent less time with the negative people in her life.

A year later, she was down nearly sixty pounds, and knew for the first time in her life that she would never go back to being overweight again.

In many ways, optimism is like exercise.

It's a fundamentally healthy habit that can enhance every aspect of our lives. It provides resilience in the face of setbacks, protects our self-image and prevents self-sabotage, and prompts us to take credit when we succeed and deflect the burden of blame when we fail. But if we embrace it too enthusiastically, it can become counterproductive and even dangerous.

Optimism can encourage big thinking and ambitious goal setting, but it can also beguile us into underestimating effort, obstacles, and opponents. It can encourage spirited action, but it can also embolden us to the point of recklessness. It can encourage buoyancy, but it can also distort reality, even to the point of delusion.

All this is why we want an abundance of optimism in our lives, but not too much. Enough to keep us uplifted and looking upward, but not so much that we float into the clouds and lose track of what's up and down.

Recommended Reading
Positivity by Barbara Fredrickson

Do This Now

For the next several minutes, consider your body, inside and out, and write down answers to the following questions:

- What is right about my body?
- What am I okay with?
- What can I enjoy, admire, and even celebrate?

Next, reflect on what things might be like if your body didn't possess these positive qualities. What if they were taken away? How would this impact your life? Write down your answers.

Now write down an example of a time where you told yourself a pessimistic story about something negative that happened in your life.

How could you have formed an optimistic story instead? What might that story have looked like? Write it down.

Next, take one of your "big five" goals you wrote down at the end of Chapter 4, and conduct a "premortem" on it.

Here's a refresher on how:

Start by assuming that the undertaking has failed spectacularly. Then, over the next few minutes, write down every reason you can think of for the failure, and pay special attention to the kinds of things you might not want to consider as potential problems due to ego or, if you're in a group, impoliteness.

Assuming you have failed spectacularly at the goal you've chosen to analyze, write down every reason you can think of for the failure.

Now, in light of the pitfalls you've uncovered, generate and write down ideas for how you can minimize their likelihood of occurring or avoid them altogether.

CHAPTER FOURTEEN

Beware the "Self-Made" Myth

"I've learned that you shouldn't go through life with a catcher's mitt on both hands; you need to be able to throw something back."
—Maya Angelou

The Grant Study is one of the longest-running observational studies ever conducted.

It began in 1938 and has followed the lives of 268 Harvard undergraduate men for seventy-five years, measuring an astonishing number of psychological, anthropological, and physical traits, ranging from personality type to IQ, drinking habits, family relationships, and even "hanging length of his scrotum." (You never know what the data might reveal!)

This project was undertaken to determine what factors contribute most to human well-being, and George Vaillant, who directed the study for over forty-two years, published its most striking findings in his 2012 book *Triumphs of Experience*.

Among them are the obvious (alcoholism is incredibly destructive), the encouraging (moderately intelligent people have the same earning potential as highly intelligent folk), and the peculiar (politically left-leaning men tend to be more sexually active later in life).

The crown jewel of the entire endeavor, however, is the single factor that appears to be most powerfully correlated with flourishing: the warmth of your relationships.

"The seventy-five years and twenty million dollars expended on the Grant Study points . . . to a straightforward five-word conclusion," Vaillant says. "'Happiness is love. Full stop.'"

The men who scored highest on measurements of "warm relationships" earned more money than those who scored lowest, achieved more professional acclaim, and experienced less anxiety, dementia, and other disorders.

Vaillant's best advice to all of us who want to be healthy and happy, then, is to cultivate positive and meaningful relationships.

This conclusion has been supported by other research as well. For example, a study conducted by scientists at the University of Michigan looked at two hundred seventy thousand people in nearly one hundred countries, and found that while both family and friends are associated with happiness and better health, as people got older, the health benefits remained only in those who had strong friendships.[1]

It turns out Vaillant's guidance is pretty good fitness advice too, because your relationships can also significantly impact your diet and exercise habits.

In one study conducted by scientists at Harvard University, a person's chances of becoming obese increased by 57 percent if they had a friend who had become obese. Among pairs of siblings, if one became obese, the chance that the other would become obese increased by 40 percent. If one spouse became obese, the likelihood that the other would become obese increased by 37 percent.[2]

This phenomenon cuts the other way too. In her 2017 book *The Transformational Consumer*, Tara-Nicholle Nelson shared the following data from her time working at MyFitnessPal:

- Users who shared their food diary with friends lost twice as much weight as those who didn't.
- Users who had ten or more friends in the app lost four times as much weight as users who went it alone.
- Fifty-six percent of users said they preferred to exercise with others because it made them more likely to show up and work hard.

Even Arnold Schwarzenegger has said he couldn't have made it as a bodybuilder, actor, businessman, and politician without all the help he received from many people at every point in his journey.

"You can call me Arnold. You can call me Schwarzenegger. You can call me the Austrian Oak. You can call me Schwarzy. You can call me Arnie. But don't ever, ever call me the self-made man," he said in his 2017 commencement address at the University of Houston. "The whole concept of the self-made man or woman is a myth."[3]

He went on in that speech to share parts of his story that you don't hear in motivational monologues and biographical sketches.

Arnold's mother tutored him through school, his father taught him how to play sports and develop discipline, a lifeguard taught him how to do his first chin-up, coaches taught him weightlifting and powerlifting, fitness magnate Joe Weider brought him to America and gave him a place to live, men and women patiently gave him acting, voice, English, speech, and accent removal lessons, studio executives, producers, and directors found roles for him, teams of specialists worked tirelessly to make him look and sound great on the silver screen, and Jay Leno helped him announce his candidacy for the governorship on his late-night show.

"So, this is why it is important for all of us to recognize, and this is why I tell you, on every step of the way I had help," Arnold said. "And the reason why I want you to understand that is because as soon as you understand that you are here because of a lot of help, then you also understand that now is time to help others. That's what this is all about. You've got to help others. Don't just think about yourself. Help others."

I couldn't agree more. You wouldn't be reading this book if I hadn't received the help, directly or indirectly, of literally thousands of people—researchers, writers, readers, followers, colleagues, friends, and family, to name a few—to say nothing of all the people who have helped me get into a position where I could write the book in the first place. I scoff at the notion of being a self-made man. I was taught at an early age that no matter what you want to do, don't try to go it alone. You won't get very far.

"Most of us assume that people achieve success and then start giving back," Dr. Adam Grant said in an 2013 interview in *Scientific American*. "But what if the opposite is true? Could it be that giving first actually leads people to succeed later?"[4]

Dr. Grant provides a thoughtful answer to that question in his 2013 book *Give and Take*, where he explains why some of the most successful people, in not just business but life in general, are in fact classic "givers"—people who genuinely try to help those around them.

Use this insight to your advantage. Every aspiration of yours is going to require help from others, which means you will always have opportunities to give back. If you can find joy in that reciprocation and strive to give more than you take, you will become what Dr. Grant refers to as a "giver," and your chances of personal success and satisfaction will increase markedly.

An easy way to incorporate this into your daily routine is to recruit a friend or friends to work out with you. You will all benefit from this in several ways:

- You'll be there to spot each and other and help improve each other's technique.
- You'll provide each other with accountability and external motivation.
- You'll help each other stick to your diet and exercise programs better.[5]
- You'll help each other push harder in your workouts.[6]
- You'll help each other have more fun in your workouts.[7]

Another easy way to do more giving is to remember that it doesn't require that we try to become Mother Theresa or Mahatma Gandhi. It simply means finding ways to add value to others' lives, and it doesn't have to cost more than five minutes of our time.

As Oprah Winfrey once said: "No gesture is too small when done with gratitude."

This can also have a ripple effect in your life by encouraging the people you touch to do the same for the people they can touch, who can be encouraged to do the same, and so on.

What could these "five-minute favors" be? Whatever people might find helpful!

For example, you could . . .

- Share a useful book recommendation.
- Introduce them to someone who might be able to help them.

- Strike up a conversation with the person at the social gathering nobody is talking to.
- Send a handwritten note to thank them for something they did, even if it's just being a good friend, teacher, boss, or mentor.
- Compliment them on something they did well.
- Share, comment, or retweet something of theirs on a social network.
- Offer feedback or a testimonial on a product or service.

You get the idea. The possibilities are endless!

Recommended Reading

Give and Take by Adam Grant

Do This Now

Your mission is to do seven "five-minute favors" for people you care about over the next seven days, with no strings attached or repayment expected.

Think of seven such favors you could do, and write them down.

Then do one favor per day for the next seven days.

CHAPTER FIFTEEN

Farewell . . . For Now

"It is not our memories but the person we have become because of those past experiences thtat we should treasure."
—*Marie Kondo*

L ittle in life is more satisfying than setting daunting goals and then doing whatever it takes to make them a reality. This is when we're at our best—when we're pushing ourselves beyond our present capabilities and comfort zones to do things that expand our perceptions of what is possible.

I hope that as you close this book, you decide to embrace and embody this philosophy not only in the gym, but in other areas of your life as well. I hope my writing helps you wake every day and decide to do the hard things that will make you proud. I hope you can return regularly to these pages for inspiration and determination, and especially when you need it most. I hope that one day, as you look back on everything you did to reach a level you now only dream of, you'll say this book had something to do with it.

Remember that the real fun begins when you turn the ink

on the pages into actions in your own life. Where you are now is a result of who you were, but where you go from here and ultimately end up depends solely on who you decide to be from this moment forward.

To help you get started, I've put together a package of bonus material that will help you get more out of what you've just read, and implement the key principles and practices discussed in this book.

You can get instant access to everything at www.workout-motivationbook.com/bonus and get started right away. Yes, tomorrow can be a day that you will remember as the day when you took the first fateful step toward a new you.

Or you could put down this book right now, shove your ambitions into a memory hole, tell yourself that everything is fine the way it is, and just keep doing what you're doing. Denial is nothing if not calming, but know this: you can only ignore the truth for so long before it sucker punches you in the gut.

As difficult as it is, the sooner we face our weaknesses and shortcomings and brainstorm ways to eliminate or circumvent them, the faster we can get to where we really want to be.

So, the choice is up to you. If you're one of the brave few who chooses the red pill, you're in for an adventure, and if there's anything I can do to support you, please let me know. My goal is to help you reach your goals faster, and if we work together as a team, we can and will succeed.

Here's how we can connect:

- Facebook: www.facebook.com/muscleforlifefitness
- Twitter: www.twitter.com/muscleforlife
- Instagram: www.instagram.com/muscleforlifefitness

And last but not least, my website is www.muscleforlife.com, and if you want to write me, my email address is mike@muscleforlife.com. (Keep in mind that I get a lot of emails every day, so it may take a week or so for me to get back to you.)

Also, if you've gotten anything from this book and are better off in any way from reading it, please pass it on to someone you love. Let them borrow your copy or, better yet, get them their own as a gift and say, "I love and appreciate you and want to help you live your best life, so I got you this. Read it."

My personal mission is to get this information into as many hands as possible, and I simply can't do that without your help. So please spread the word.

Thank you so much. I hope to hear from you soon, and I wish you the best.

Would You Do Me a Favor?

Thank you for reading my book. I hope that you're able to use what I've written to look, feel, and live better than you ever have before.

I have a small favor to ask.

Would you mind taking a minute to write a blurb on Amazon about this book? I check all my reviews, and I love to get feedback. (That's the real pay for my work—knowing that I'm helping people.)

Thanks again!

Free Bonus Material (Guides, Tools, and More!)

Thanks so much for reading *The Little Black Book of Workout Motivation*.

I hope you found it insightful, inspiring, and entertaining, and I hope it helps you reach your health and fitness goals faster.

I want to make sure that you get as much value from this book as possible, so I've put together a number of additional free resources to help you, including:

- A savable, shareable, printable quickstart guide with all of the book's key takeaways, exercises, action items, and checklists.
- A list of my favorite tools for getting and staying motivated and on track inside and outside of the gym.
- Three bonus chapters on the beauty and power of difficulty, how to engineer your environment so you need less motivation, and how to use gratitude to feel less stressed and depressed, reduce the risk of chronic disease, sleep better, and more.
- My most-recommended books for building a better body and life.

- Three interviews with thought leaders Stephen Guise, James Clear, and Mark Murphy on the topics of habit formation, goal setting and accomplishment, environment design, and more.

To get instant access to all of that (plus an additional surprise gift), go here now:

www.workoutmotivationbook.com/bonus

Other Books by Michael Matthews

Bigger Leaner Stronger: The Simple Science of Building the Ultimate Male Body

Thinner Leaner Stronger: The Simple Science of Building the Ultimate Female Body

The Shredded Chef: 120 Recipes for Building Muscle, Getting Lean, and Staying Healthy

CARDIO SUCKS: The Simple Science of Losing Fat Fast...Not Muscle

Bibliography

12 Rules for Life: An Antidote to Chaos
by Jordan B. Peterson

Total Recall: My Unbelievably True Life Story
by Arnold Schwarzenegger

The Magic of Thinking Big
by David Schwartz

Hagakure: The Secret Wisdom of the Samurai
by Yamamoto Tsunetomo and translated by
Alexander Bennett

To Sell Is Human: The Surprising Truth About Moving Others
by Dan Pink

Rethinking Positive Thinking: Inside the New Science of Motivation
by Gabriele Oettingen

The Marshmallow Test: Mastering Self-Control
by Walter Mischel

Thinking, Fast and Slow
by Daniel Kahneman

Willpower: Rediscovering the Greatest Human Strength
by Roy F. Baumeister and John Tierney

Principles: Life and Work
by Ray Dalio

The Talent Code: Greatness Isn't Born. It's Grown. Here's How.
by Daniel Coyle

Do the Work
by Steven Pressfield

It Works: The Famous Little Red Book That Makes Your Dreams Come True!
by RHJ

The War of Art
by Steven Pressfield

The Motivation Myth
by Jeff Haden

The Subtle Art of Not Giving a F*ck: The Counterintuitive Approach to Living a Good Life
by Mark Manson

Hard Goals
by Mark Murphy

Mornings on Horseback: The Story of an Extraordinary Family, a Vanished Way of Life, and the Unique Child Who Became Theodore Roosevelt
by David McCullough

Alexander the Great
by Philip Freeman

Elon Musk: Tesla, SpaceX, and the Quest for a Fantastic Future
by Ashlee Vance

Titan: The Life of John D. Rockefeller, Sr
by Ron Chernow

Leonardo da Vinci
by Walter Isaacson

Stumbling on Happiness
by Daniel Gilbert

Rapt: Attention and the Focused Life
by Winifred Gallagher

Happiness: Unlocking the Mysteries of Psychological Wealth
by Ed Diener and Robert Biswas-Diener

Learned Optimism: How to Change Your Mind and Your Life
by Martin Seligman

The Happiness Advantage: How a Positive Brain Fuels Success in Work and Life
by Shawn Achor

Self Analysis
by L. Ron Hubbard

Positivity: Top-Notch Research Reveals the Upward Spiral That Will Change Your Life
by Barbara Fredrickson

Gratitude Works!: A 21-Day Program for Creating Emotional Prosperity
by Robert A. Emmons

Flourish: A Visionary New Understanding of Happiness and Well-being
by Martin Seligman

Peak Performance: Elevate Your Game, Avoid Burnout, and Thrive with the New Science of Success
by Brad Stulberg and Steve Magness

Living with a SEAL: 31 Days Training with the Toughest Man on the Planet
by Jesse Itzler

A Complaint Free World: How to Stop Complaining and Start Enjoying the Life You Always Wanted
by Will Bowen

Bigger Leaner Stronger: The Simple Science of Building the Ultimate Male Body
by Michael Matthews

Thinner Leaner Stronger: The Simple Science of Building the Ultimate Female Body
by Michael Matthews

Meditations: A New Translation
by Marcus Aurelius and translated by Gregory Hays

The Power of Intuition: How to Use Your Gut Feelings to Make Better Decisions at Work
by Gary Klein

The Gulag Archipelago
by Aleksandr Solzhenitsyn

The 33 Strategies of War
by Robert Greene

Triumphs of Experience
by George Vaillant

The Transformational Consumer: Fuel a Lifelong Love Affair with Your Customers by Helping Them Get Healthier, Wealthier, and Wiser
by Tara–Nicholle Nelson

Give and Take: Why Helping Others Drives Our Success
by Adam Grant

Make Your Bed
by William H. McRaven

References

Section 1: Cultivating the Right Mindset

THE GREAT ART OF SACRIFICE

1.   Mischel W, Shoda Y, Rodriguez MI. (1989). Delay of
     gratification in children. *Science*, 244(4907):933–938.
     doi:10.1126/SCIENCE.2658056.
     Ayduk, O., Mendoza-Denton, R., Mischel, W., Downey,
     G., Peake, P. K., & Rodriguez, M. (2000). Regulating
     the interpersonal self: strategic self-regulation for
     coping with rejection sensitivity. *Journal of Personality
     and Social Psychology*, 79(5), 776–792. Schlam TR,
     Wilson NL, Shoda Y, Mischel W, Ayduk O. Preschoolers'
     delay of gratification predicts their body mass
     30 years later. *J Pediatr.* 2013;162(1):90–93. doi:10.1016/j.
     jpeds.2012.06.049.
     Shoda Y, Mischel W, Peake PK. Predicting Adolescent
     Cognitive and Self-Regulatory Competencies From
     Preschool Delay of Gratification: Identifying Diagnostic
     Conditions. *Dev Psychol.* 1990;26(6):978–986.
2.   Martijn C, Tenbült P, Merckelbach H, Dreezens E,
     de Vries NK. Getting A Grip on Ourselves: Challenging
     Expectancies About Loss of Energy After
     Self-Control. *Soc Cogn.* 2002;20(6):441–460. doi:10.1521/
     soco.20.6.441.22978.
3.   Job, V., Dweck, C. S., & Walton, G. M. (2010). Ego
     Depletion—Is It All in Your Head? *Psychological Science*,
     21(11), 1686–1693. https://doi.

org/10.1177/0956797610384745.

4. Duckworth, A. L., Gendler, T. S., & Gross, J. (2016). Situational Strategies for Self-Control. *Perspec tives on Psychological Science : A Journal of the Associa tion for Psychological Science*, 11(1), 35–55. https://doi. org/10.1177/1745691615623247.

5. Zajonc, R. B. (1968). Attitudinal effects of mere exposure. *Journal of Personality and Social Psycholog*y, 9(2, Pt.2), 1–27. https://doi.org/10.1037/h0025848.

6. Lally, P., van Jaarsveld, C. H. M., Potts, H. W. W., & Wardle, J. (2010). How are habits formed: Modelling habit formation in the real world. *European Journal of Social Psychology*, 40(6), 998–1009. https://doi.org/10.1002/ ejsp.674.

7. Painter, J. E., Wansink, B., & Hieggelke, J. B. (2002). How visibility and convenience influence candy consumption. *Appetite*, 38(3), 237–238. https://doiorg/10.1006/appe.2002.0485.

8. Hunter, J. A., Hollands, G. J., Couturier, D.-L., & Marteau, T. M. (2018). Effect of snack-food proximity on intake in general population samples with higher and lower cognitive resource. *Appetite*, 121, 337–347. https://doi. org/10.1016/j.appet.2017.11.101.

9. McClure, S. M., Ericson, K. M., Laibson, D. I., Loewenstein, G., & Cohen, J. D. (2007). Time Discount ing for Primary Rewards. *Journal of Neuroscience*, 27(21), 5796–5804. https://doi.org/10.1523/JNEUROSCI.4246- 06.2007.

10. Matthews, M. (2018). I Took Cold Showers for a Year and Here's What Happened | Muscle For Life.

11. Bilton, N. (2014). Disruptions: For a Restful Night, Make Your Smartphone Sleep on the Couch - The New York Times.

Gnambs, T., & Appel, M. (2018). Narcissism and Social Networking Behavior: A Meta-Analysis. *Journal of Personality*, 86(2), 200–212. https://doi.org/10.1111/jopy.12305.

Lup, K., Trub, L., & Rosenthal, L. (2015). Instagram #Instasad?: Exploring Associations Among Instagram Use, Depressive Symptoms, Negative Social Comparison, and Strangers Followed. *Cyberpsychology, Behavior, and Social Networking*, 18(5), 247–252. https://doi.org/10.1089/cyber.2014.0560.

12. Maybin, S. (2017). Busting the attention span myth - BBC News.

13. Ophir, E., Nass, C., & Wagner, A. D. (2009). Cognitive control in media multitaskers. *Proceedings of the National Academy of Sciences of the United States of America*, 106(37), 15583–15587. https://doi.org/10.1073/pnas.0903620106

THE TROUBLE WITH WAITING FOR PERFECT

1. Wicker, A. W. (1969). Attitudes versus Actions: The Relationship of Verbal and Overt Behavioral Responses to Attitude Objects. *Journal of Social Issues*, 25(4), 41–78. https://doi.org/10.1111/j.1540-4560.1969.tb00619.x.

Section 2: Setting Goals

THE WRONG WAY AND RIGHT WAY TO SET GOALS

1. Schippers, M. C., Scheepers, A. W. A., & Peterson, J. B. (2015). A scalable goal-setting intervention closes

both the gender and ethnic minority achievement gap. *Palgrave Communications*, 1(1), 15014. https://doi.org/10.1057/palcomms.2015.14.

HOW TO NOT SUCK AT ACHIEVING YOUR GOALS

1. Senay, I., Albarracín, D., & Noguchi, K. (2010). Motivating goal-directed behavior through introspective self-talk: the role of the interrogative form of simple future tense. *Psychological Science*, 21(4), 499–504. https://doi.org/10.1177/0956797610364751.

2. Milne, S., Orbell, S., & Sheeran, P. (2002). Combining motivational and volitional interven   tions to promote exercise participation: Protection motivation theory and implementation intentions. *British Journal of Health Psychology*, 7(2), 163–184. https://doi.org/10.1348/135910702169420.

3. Rise, J., Thompson, M., & Verplanken, B. (2003). Measuring implementation intentions in the context of the theory of planned behavior. *Scandinavian Journal of Psychology*, 44(2), 87–95.
   Prestwich, A., Lawton, R., & Conner, M. (2003). The use of implementation intentions and the decision balance sheet in promoting exercise behaviour. *Psychology & Health*, 18(6), 707–721. https://doi.org/10.1080/0887044031 0001594493.
   Orbell, S., Hodgkins, S., & Sheeran, P. (1997). Implementation Intentions and the Theory of Planned Behavior. *Personality and Social Psychology Bulletin*, 23(9), 945–954. https://doi.org/10.1177/0146167297239004
   Verplanken, B., & Faes, S. (1999). Good intentions, bad habits, and effects of forming implementation intentions on healthy eating. *European Journal of Social Psychology*,

29(5–6), 591–604.

Teng, Y., & Mak, W. W. S. (2011). The role of planning and self-efficacy in condom use among men who have sex with men: An application of the Health Action Process Approach model. *Health Psychology*, 30(1), 119–128. https://doi.org/10.1037/a0022023

Griva, F., Anagnostopoulos, F., & Madoglou, S. (2010). Mammography Screening and the Theory of Planned Behavior: Suggestions Toward an Extended Model of Prediction. *Women & Health*, 49(8), 662–681. https://doi.org/10.1080/03630240903496010.

Roncancio, A. M., Ward, K. K., Sanchez, I. A., Cano, M. A., Byrd, T. L., Vernon, S. W., … Fernandez, M. E. (2015). Using the Theory of Planned Behavior to Understand Cervical Cancer Screening Among Latinas. *Health Education & Behavior : The Official Publication of the Society for Public Health Education*, 42(5), 621–626. https://doi.org/10.1177/1090198115571364.

Pawlak, R., Brown, D., Meyer, M. K., Connell, C., Yadrick, K., Johnson, J. T., & Blackwell, A. (2008). Theory of Planned Behavior and Multivitamin Supplement Use in Caucasian College Females. *The Journal of Primary Prevention*, 29(1), 57–71. https://doi.org/10.1007/s10935-008-0127-y.

Cooke, R., Dahdah, M., Norman, P., & French, D. P. (2016). How well does the theory of planned behaviour predict alcohol consumption? A systematic review and meta-analysis. *Health Psychology Review*, 10(2), 148–167. https://doi.org/10.1080/17437199.2014.947547.

Godin, G., & Kok, G. (1996). The Theory of Planned Behavior: A Review of its Applications to Health-Relat ed Behaviors. *American Journal of Health Promotion*, 11(2), 87–98. https://doi.org/10.4278/0890-1171-11.2.87.

4. Kappes, A., Singmann, H., & Oettingen, G. (2012). Mental contrasting instigates goal pursuit by linking obstacles of reality with instrumental behavior. *Journal of Experimental Social Psychology*, 48(4), 811–818. https://doi.org/10.1016/J.JESP.2012.02.002.

5. Gollwitzer PM, Sheeran P, Michalski V, Seifert AE. When Intentions Go Public. Psychol Sci. 2009;20(5):612–618. doi:10.1111/j.1467-9280.2009.02336.x.

6. Matthews, G. (n.d.). Study focuses on strategies for achieving goals, resolutions — Dominican University of California.

7. Tannenbaum, M. B., Hepler, J., Zimmerman, R. S., Saul, L., Jacobs, S., Wilson, K., & Albarracín,D. (2015). Appealing to fear: A meta-analysis of fear appeal effectiveness and theories. *Psychological Bulletin*, 141(6), 1178–1204. https://doi.org/10.1037/a0039729.

Section 3: Doing the Work

EXCUSES OR PROGRESS: CHOOSE ONE

1. Goleman, D. (1984). Excuses: New Theory Defines Their Role in Life - The New York Times.

2. Stocks, A., & April, K. A. (2012). Locus of control and subjective well-being - a cross-cultural study. *Problems and Perspectives in Management*, 10(1).

Section 4: Staying on Top

THE CURSE OF COMPLAINING

1. Lohr, J. M., Olatunji, B. O., Baumeister, R. F., & Bushman, B. J. (2007). The psychology of anger venting and empirically supported alternatives that do no harm. *The Scientific Review of Mental Health Practice: Objective Investigations of Controversial and Unorthodox Claims in Clinical Psychology, Psychiatry, and Social Work*, 5(1), 53–64.
    Wojciszke, B., Baryla, W., Szymków-Sudziarska, A., Parzuchowski, M., & Kowalczyk, K. (2009). Saying is experiencing: Affective consequences of complaining and affirmation. *Polish Psychological Bulletin*, 40(2), 74–84. https://doi.org/10.2478/s10059-009-0008-0.
    Kowalski, R. M. (1996). Complaints and complaining: Functions, antecedents, and consequences. Psycholog ical Bulletin, 119(2), 179–196. https://doi.org/10.1037/0033-2909.119.2.179.
    Lehmann-Willenbrock, N., & Kauffeld, S. (2010). The downside of communication: Complaining cycles in group discussions. *In S. Schuman (Ed.), The handbook for working with difficult groups: How they are difficult, why they are difficult, what you can do*, 33–54.
2. Crum, A. J., Salovey, P., & Achor, S. (2013). Rethink ing stress: The role of mindsets in determining the stress response. *Journal of Personality and Social Psychology*, 104(4), 716–733. https://doi.org/10.1037/a0031201.
3. Keller, A., Litzelman, K., Wisk, L. E., Maddox, T., Cheng, E. R., Creswell, P. D., & Witt, W. P. (2012). Does the perception that stress affects health matter? The

association with health and mortality. *Health Psychology : Official Journal of the Division of Health Psychology, American Psychological Association*, 31(5), 677–684. https://doi.org/10.1037/a0026743.

4. Brooks, A. W. (2014). Get excited: Reappraising pre-per formance anxiety as excitement. *Journal of Experimental Psychology: General*, 143(3), 1144–1158. https://doi. org/10.1037/a0035325.

THE POSITIVITY PARADOX

1. Sharot, T. (2011). The optimism bias. *Current Biology*, 21(23), R941–R945. https://doi.org/10.1016/J. CUB.2011.10.030.

2. Hmieleski, K. M., & Baron, R. A. (2009). Entrepreneurs' Optimism And New Venture Performance: A Social Cognitive Perspective. *Academy of Management Journal*, 52(3), 473–488. https://doi.org/10.5465/ AMJ.2009.41330755.
Parke, J., Griffiths, M. D., & Parke, A. (2007). Positive Thinking Among Slot Machine Gamblers: A Case of Maladaptive Coping? *International Journal of Mental Health and Addiction*, 5(1), 39–52. https://doi.org/10.1007/ s11469-006-9049-1.
Verkuil, P. R., Seligman, M., & Kang, T. (2000). Counter ing Lawyer Unhappiness: Pessimism, Decision Latitude and the Zero-Sum Dilemma. *SSRN Electronic Journal*. https://doi.org/10.2139/ssrn.241942.

3. Verkuil, P. R., Seligman, M., & Kang, T. (2000). Counter ing Lawyer Unhappiness: Pessimism, Decision Latitude and the Zero-Sum Dilemma. *SSRN Electronic Journal*. https://doi.org/10.2139/ssrn.241942.

4. The Science Behind the Smile - Harvard Business Review. (2012).

5. Kahneman, D., & Deaton, A. (2010). High income improves evaluation of life but not emotional well-be ing. *Proceedings of the National Academy of Sciences of the United States of America*, 107(38), 16489–16493. https://doi.org/10.1073/pnas.1011492107.

6. Brickman, P., Coates, D., & Janoff-Bulman, R. (1978). Lottery winners and accident victims: Is happiness relative? *Journal of Personality and Social Psychology*, 36(8), 917-927. http://dx.doi.org/10.1037/0022-3514.36.8.917.

7. Wilson Daniel T Gilbert, T. D. (2000). Affective Forecast ing. *Advances in Experimental Social Psychology*.

8. Stutzer, A., & Frey, B. S. (n.d.). Stress That Doesn't Pay: The Commuting Paradox. *The Scandinavian Journal of Economics*. https://doi.org/10.2307/25195346.
    Hershfield, H. E., Mogilner, C., & Barnea, U. (2016). People Who Choose Time Over Money Are Happier. *Social Psychological and Personality Science*, 7(7), 697–706. https://doi.org/10.1177/1948550616649239.
    Thaler RH. Misbehaving: The Making of Behavioral Economics. 1st ed. W.W. Norton & Company; 2015.

9. Stickgold, R., Malia, A., Maguire, D., Roddenberry, D., & O'Connor, M. (2000). Replaying the game: hypnagogic images in normals and amnesics. *Science* (New York, N.Y.), 290(5490), 350–353. https://doi.org/10.1126/SCIENCE.290.5490.350.

10. Earling, A. (March 21–28, 1996). The Tetris effect: Do computer games fry your brain? Philadelphia City Paper.

11. Peterson, C., Seligman, M. E., & Vaillant, G. E. (1988). Pessimistic explanatory style is a risk factor for physical illness: a thirty-five-year longitudinal study. *Journal of Personality and Social Psychology*, 55(1), 23–27.

12. Seligman, M. (2006). *Learned Optimism: How to Change*

Your Mind and Your Life. New York, NY: Vintage Books.

13. Klein, G. (2007). Performing a Project Premortem – Harvard Business Review.

14. Mitchell, D. J., Edward Russo, J., & Pennington, N. (1989). Back to the future: Temporal perspective in the explana tion of events. *Journal of Behavioral Decision Making*, 2(1), 25–38. https://doi.org/10.1002/bdm.3960020103.

BEWARE THE "SELF-MADE" MYTH

1. Chopik, W. J. (2017). Associations among relational values, support, health, and well-being across the adult lifespan. *Personal Relationships*, 24(2), 408–422. https://doi.org/10.1111/pere.12187.

2. Christakis, N. A., & Fowler, J. H. (2007). The Spread of Obesity in a Large Social Network over 32 Years. *New England Journal of Medicine*, 357(4), 370–379. https://doi.org/10.1056/NEJMsa066082.

3. Arnold Schwarzenegger at the University of Houston | Time. (2017).

4. Cook, G. (2013). The Secret to Success Is Giving, Not Taking – *Scientific American*.

5. Wing, R. R., & Jeffery, R. W. (1999). Benefits of recruiting participants with friends and increasing social support for weight loss and maintenance. *Journal of Consulting and Clinical Psychology*, 67(1), 132–138.

6. Feltz, D. L., Kerr, N. L., & Irwin, B. C. (2011). Buddy Up: The Köhler Effect Applied to Health Games. *Journal of Sport and Exercise Psychology*, 33(4), 506–526. https://doi.org/10.1123/jsep.33.4.506.

7. Dunton, G. F., Liao, Y., Intille, S., Huh, J., & Leventhal, A. (2015). Momentary assessment of contextual influences on affective response during physical activity. *Health Psychology*, 34(12), 1145–1153. https://doi.org/10.1037/hea0000223.